MW00425806

LAST SOUL STANDING

Surviving My Last Surviving Relative

Marilyn Poscic

http://www.marilynposcic.com

ISBN: 978-1479396092

First Printing, 2012

Published by 102nd Place, LLC

Scottsdale, AZ

Printed in the United States of America

Table of Contents

Prelude

I wish to dedicate this book to Margaret Lawrence, my Mother, Howard Lawrence, my Father, and Eric Lawrence, my Brother, whom I love dearly and who suffered greatly in the last years of their lives. Their courage and abundant love for everyone and everything continues to be my inspiration. This book was written to help the millions of you out there who are going through, are about to go through, will go through, or have already been through, the experiences you are about to read. It is about encountering a medical turmoil with a loved one, no matter how that loved one relates to you. The insights and actions may apply no matter what the medical condition and no matter the age. Don't think that crises only affect the old. Oh No!

Please don't be under the misconception that this will never happen to you or those you love. Mainly though, don't be under the mindset if something traumatic does happen, that there are professionals out there to help and guide you. Yes there are. But you have to know how to find them, what questions to ask, and what actions to take. They cannot make decisions for you. Many professionals are so busy they do not have the time to sit down and discuss all of the options. Many don't care and others can't advise due to legal or financial reasons.

As you will read, in my life there were various types of tragedies that struck my family, which of course affected me. The last one though was a real awakening for me. I had been an x-ray technician for over 20 years, had worked in a hospital lab for 5 years, and had worked as a back office nurse for over 10 years.

After my brother's passing in 1995, I started wondering what happens when we die. Why him and why now? I read a book called "Embraced by the Light" by Betty J. Eadie which answered some of my questions but raised even more. In 1998 I saw a world renowned Angel Messenger in Scottsdale, AZ. At that time I had never heard of an Angel Messenger, especially in human form but she was able to answer more of my questions. She also enlightened me to the world of Angels and communicating with deceased loved ones.

I retained knowledge from this seminar, not realizing a year later my own spiritual gifts would awaken and I would start communicating with Angels and those who had passed. I now do this on a professional level helping others to find answers. But at the time it got me thinking. If I was blindsided by the events I am about to recount, with all of my knowledge, both medically and metaphysically, what happens to the people out there who have no medical or spiritual knowledge, or personal experience with the incapacitation and then death of a loved one?

While going through my mother's tragedy I kept saying, when the dust settles for me I am going to write a book to help enlighten people. I have put together this book, based on my true life experiences. I have also given helpful reference guides as to which professionals you can turn to along with questions and actions that can be taken.

I feel with my whole heart that if this book helps just one person, I am blessed. If that one person shares with another, then they share with another, then they share..... to reach out to help hundreds, thousands, millions, then we are all blessed.

I wish you all many blessings of happiness, healthfulness, love and a greater enlightenment about the medical process and the benefits of the spiritual world!!

Marilyn Poscic

Togetherness

Mom was 87 years young. She hadn't been to a doctor in over four years and then only because she had shingles. And before that - who knows? I remember taking her to the doctor for a physical, perhaps six or seven years earlier. The doctor told her she was in good health and to come back when she got sick. She took no medication. This was a good thing because we both believed in trying everything natural as we felt prescription medication often did more harm than good. Mom could walk and talk and had a memory like an elephant. Trust me I know. Some things I wished she had or could forget!

Margaret loved life. She loved to have a good time. I remember her laughing; sometimes laughing so hard she peed in her pants. And she liked to party, meaning drinking beer, sometimes rum or vodka, a little Kahlua in her coffee. Now don't get me wrong. She didn't drink all the time or every day. But she loved having people over, laughing, going out, and gambling. You know typical 87 year old, right? Not! Everyone has their individuality!

After the passing of my brother in 1995, I began to wonder what happens after we die, or as I now like to say, we pass. A friend of mine gave me a book to read, "Embraced by the Light", by Betty J. Eadie. That book answered some questions for me but raised even more. In 1998, another friend of mine took me to see Doreen Virtue, a world renowned Angel Messenger. At that time I had never heard of Angel Messengers but did know and understand to some degree the role of a psychic. Mom and I discussed these thoughts and feelings from time to time. She did believe in psychics, but more importantly, she believed in God and Angels, although we were not religious. Margaret believed strongly, that my brother spoke to her from time to time, and visited her often through a butterfly on her front porch.

In 1999, while I was in Boston for four months opening kiosks in malls with an all-natural dietary supplement, I had my own spiritual awakening. The manager who had come with me was very psychic but extremely scared of it. She saw a big white light around me and told me so. It frightened me, so I called upon Arc Angel Michael to protect me. This is what I had learned to do from Doreen, the Angel Messenger. My manager was able to see Michael as well! The two of us started experimenting with these possibilities for many nights. Then one night she was able to see my deceased brother, Eric, describe him in detail and deliver a message to me. In turn, I was able to see her deceased son, describe him in detail as well and deliver a message from him!

Upon returning to Phoenix and seeing friends I had not seen in at least four months, I was able to see either Angels or deceased loved ones around them and deliver messages. This new ability still scared me and I spent many hours discussing my thoughts and feelings with my mom. I know in my heart she believed me because I was raised not to lie. I know she believed in other people who did this, but I think she had a hard time comprehending and accepting that I now had "abilities" as well. Little did either one of us know that later I would become a professional Angel Messenger and Medium.

Mom loved interacting with people, both in a socializing, party atmosphere and in helping by lending an ear, giving a shoulder to lean on, or giving advice when warranted. But the most special person in her life was me. We loved each other greatly.

That's not to say we didn't have our moments. You know that mother/daughter thing. In addition to all the great fun good times, there were also times when she would get mad at me. She would get that stubborn streak going and then not talk to me for extended periods of time. But we always made up. Trust me. You must do this. As you will see, you just never know.

We loved doing things together like entertaining on her front porch. In fact two days before "s" day, we had several people over celebrating a good friend's 90th birthday. We'd do lunch, happy hour, and shop 'til we dropped. Then there were the trips. Margaret especially liked going to Yuma, Az. We could eat, drink, gamble, and go shopping right across the border in Mexico. Perfect!

However, she was not afraid to go out by herself particularly to gamble. Until about three years ago, she would get in her car and drive to Laughlin, NV, a four hour drive, all alone. She loved to listen to her music and stop at gift shops along the way, getting to know not only the people who worked in those shops but most of the employees at the casino as well. She would always make new friends everywhere she went.

Our best trip together was in May 2009, one month before the "s" day. She had accumulated enough comps to receive roundtrip airfare for two, a hotel for four nights, and of course all the food and drinks we could want at a casino in Lake Tahoe. Mom really, really wanted to go. Being a realtor in Phoenix, Az. at that time, I was hesitant. You still need money to gamble, right?

About a month before the Lake Tahoe trip she had gone to a local casino where she loved to play and often won on their butterfly slot machines. (Imagine! Was this Eric helping her?!) Before she went she talked to my deceased brother. She asked Eric, if it was meant for us to take this vacation, would he please help her make it happen? Shortly after asking, she hit a jackpot for around $1500! Mom even managed to figure out how to use her cell phone to call me and let me know we were going to Lake Tahoe because we were meant to go!

Now I had no excuses. Thank God! That was our last trip together. What a great time we had! On our first night we went to an expensive steak house in the casino. I ordered the chateaubriand, which mom had never had. She about croaked when the bill said $72! I explained, it was a complete meal for two (most dinners were around $35-$40 for one), and not to worry because she had enough comps and the casino was buying. She admitted later it was the best meal she had ever had!

On our way back to the room that night (mind you, it was around 2:00 a.m. and she's 87) I made her sit down at two slot machines. She was truly amazed since I rarely play slots. Quickly she became mortified, when she discovered they were only penny slots! I insisted on playing. We laughed so hard at these machines. We kept receiving bonuses, never knew why or how. Never did figure them out that night. But we both walked away from them with over $200 in each of our pockets.

On this special trip we truly bonded. We gambled, met new people, and we laughed so hard we peed our pants! And yes, we did come back with some of their money! Make sure you make the time to truly enjoy, bond if you will, with your loved one. You never know what lies of ahead of you. There are no "do overs" in life.

"S" Day

In June of 2009 we headed to a local casino with a friend and his wife, Steve and Kirsten, to celebrate Steve's birthday. The four of us planned on spending the night. We set off to go to our room but Mom goes in a different direction than when I normally would spend the night with her here. "I know where I'm going," she said when I questioned her on direction. After confirming with an employee just to make sure, of course she was correct! We had one cocktail in the room, and then off to the casino we went!

I always allowed mom to go wherever she wanted in a casino. She didn't like to be "hovered" around. The rest of us went to the bar for cocktails and video poker. Within 20 minutes, mom comes by waving winning tickets for around $200, thrilled and on her way to conquer yet another machine! I played tour guide with my friends, and then left them on their own.

As I started hanging around a black jack table, mind you roughly only less than one hour had transpired at this time, I got this overwhelming feeling to find mom. I located my friends, but no mom. I even asked a security person if he had seen a white haired old lady in there! His eyes had the look of a "deer in headlights," then he started laughing. Of course there's only about several hundred people that match that description in a casino!

So back to the black jack table I go. A little voice said look to your left. As I did, there was my mother on the floor! I rushed over, my heart in my throat, to see what was happening. Casino personnel and paramedics were all milling around. They explained that all they knew at this point was that she fell backward from her chair hitting her head.

Mom was totally coherent, but shaking badly and of course frightened. She said that she had sat down, gotten dizzy, and fallen backwards hitting her head. Shaking so bad myself, but having over 20 years of experience in the medical field as an x-ray technician and back office nurse, I had her start taking in deep breaths, while I tried to calm and soothe her.

The paramedics stepped in to do their evaluation. As I watched, I realized to my horror she had suffered a stroke. She kept repeating no hospital, but I calmed her down and assured her she needed to go and I would follow. They air evacuated her to a trauma hospital noted for treating stroke victims. Mind you, less than an hour ago, she was bouncing around smiling, laughing, knowing where the room was, and winning on slots but now reduced to what?

She had no use of her left side. Luckily, since she suffered her stroke in the casino she was able to receive medical treatment immediately, including getting much needed oxygen. She made it to the hospital and through the tests, only to confirm what I already knew. She had experienced a stroke. What I didn't know was that it was a massive stroke.

The doctor, given Margaret's age and small build, only gave her a 40% survival rate. Little did he know! Even if she did survive, during which the next 48 hours would be crucial, she would never regain use of her left side. Now I ask you; for a person that has been independent for 87 years, to now have to always be dependent on someone, is this living? Is this how she would want to live?

We had many conversations over the years, after watching my brother slowly die of AIDS at 34 years and my dad of Alzheimer's. We were both in agreement that if we ever became incapacitated then we didn't want to live anymore, especially if it happened at an advanced age. No life support; nothing. Mind you, these are individual choices. And although I had many years in the medical field, and we had both watched two loved ones suffer, ultimately passing after long courageous battles with life, nothing had really prepared us for what lay ahead.

The Hospital

As mom was being taken by helicopter, I was frantically driving to the hospital trying to avoid speeding tickets, with my mind racing. I walk into the Emergency Room on a Friday night in downtown Phoenix, Az. Not pretty. I finally find out which room she's in, only to discover that she's not there. Has she passed? Gone for tests? What?

I could not locate a medical professional to help me. I know they are busy, but this is my mother! Of course at this stage, you and your loved one are the only people in the world they need to pay attention to, right? After racing around, verbally attacking anyone within a two mile radius of me including picking up a clipboard and slamming it down, it was explained she was having a CT scan. So I wait, mind still racing.

After what seemed like days, but in reality only an hour or so, they wheel her back to her ER room. I look at her lying there so helpless, pale, scared, confused, with her mouth drawn and no use of her left side and tubes everywhere. Luckily I knew what the tubes were for. Would you?

How could this be happening? Just a few hours ago, we were in the casino. She was laughing, showing us to our room, winning on the slots. In other words NO warning! Now reduced to this? NO! Not my mom!

Now in comes the Doctor. Good news - the stroke affected the right side of her brain, which means her left side is paralyzed and she has limited speech abilities, but her memory is not affected. Bad news - she probably won't make it through the night. But there is that 40% chance. If she does pull through she will never be able to walk, use her left arm, or have control of her bodily functions. Is that living?

Can anyone explain to me how the "good" part is "good news"? Especially for someone who was totally independent, no medications, and no doctors in years? A woman who was still doing her own yard work, cleaning, shopping, and banking? Now lying here so scared, pale, and unable to move; looking to me for answers and to please help! I just wanted to hold her and tell her everything would be OK. This was just a bad dream. We would both wake up and be in the casino, laughing with our friends.

My legs were shaking so bad I don't know how I was able to stand there and comfort her. I just wanted to crumble, cry, run, and hide. I'd do anything to get out of this nightmare. Imagine, me of all people feeling this way. Me, this very strong, independent person was crumbling like a baby. I reprimanded myself. What good would this do for anyone if I submit to my fear and horror? I have to be strong for both of us. So I "pull up my big girl's pants," stroke her arm and pet her on the head to give as much reassurance to both of us as I can muster even though deep within my heart I know it will never be all right again.

The Doctor informs me that she will be moved to ICU. The next 48 hours are crucial. I should go home and get some rest. Seriously? Is he talking to me? I can't leave her even though deep down, I know he's right. She's so scared. There's nothing I can do. They have my contact numbers. It's all up to the medical staff, but most important, it's up to Margaret and her higher spirit.

I inform the doctor she is DNR - do not resuscitate. I have to produce the necessary paper work. Tonight? No it can wait until the morning. But it is necessary to have it as soon as possible. Great! And that might be where? Next come all the people with questions; insurance information, allergies, surgeries, doctor information, last time seen by doctor, why? Really they want me to use my brain now? I can't even find it, let alone use it! Fortunately, I had her purse. Mom was very savvy. She had all the information with her including dates of all past surgeries. Did she have a premonition and knew to carry this information with her at all times? Do you carry your information with you?

This was a great lesson to be learned. Under normal circumstances, I would have known the answers to their questions. Trust me, these were not normal circumstances. Your mind just leaves, in some cases never to be found again. Luckily, not in my case even

21

though there were days I knew it left, or I wished it would!

Now what are they asking me? I give a blank look to the person speaking to me. "What," I hear myself say. Oh now you want money before you will do anything else? Thankfully, her deductible was only $50. But yes they want their money up front. At this point I was willing to pay any amount just to make it all go away. Will it go away? Will I ever think clearly again?

Leaving

I decide to go home. Don't want to, but I know it's the right choice. Mom is in higher hands than mine. I did call upon the Angels and God for their help. Being an Angel Messenger and Medium, I know how to connect with the higher sources very well, although I must admit when things are happening to you it is extremely difficult. I ask for Mom to be in peace with no suffering and to protect, guide and comfort her.

The hospital has my contact information and all the other information they need. I don't know what lies ahead. I do know it will not do anyone any good if I become sick, exhausted, or wind up in a mental institution, since I am her last surviving relative. Steve and Kirsten, my friends who had ridden with me from the casino, spent many hours just sitting in the ER waiting room. Fortunately they were able to get in touch with their son and leave with my thanks and blessings.

Now it is just me and mom. I ask many times, do I leave or go? I think back to the classes and readings I do, teaching people that you must take care of yourself before you can take care of others. I listen to my own advice and decide to go home.

On my way, I have a complete melt down. Uncontrollable tears, sobbing, and many unpleasant words come pouring forth all while doing 70 mph. I call upon The Angels to protect me. Last thing I need is to be in or cause an accident. And they did protect me. I kid you not. Any car that seemed like it had been close to me just disappeared.

I didn't want to be alone. I called a friend, Phyllis, who just happened to be close to my house right at that time. Coincidence? I don't think so. She made a U-turn and beat me to my house. She called in the "troops"; mutual friends who came over to spend the night with me. We stayed up most of the night, laughing, drinking, talking, mostly crying, shaking; still trying to get my brain to register everything.

Then the fear factor sets in every time the phone rings. What do I do next? I am all alone. Yes I have my dear friends with me, thank God! But I wish for a spouse, significant other, sibling, child, or relative. Anyone who knew my mother and loved her as much as I did to help me with everything. But I am the last soul standing.

I know any decisions that will need to be made, will come from me alone. I love my friends, but they cannot make the decisions for me. Why couldn't I have at least one living relative to help me with the choices I knew were coming my way from all of my past experiences if she continued to survive? What if I make the wrong decision? Would I be able to live with that? I keep telling myself, I am a strong person. I know her better than anyone.

On the other side, what if I did have a whole family to deal with? Unfortunately, often when a family feels death is imminent for a loved one, money tends to become a priority. Trust me, she didn't have much but I know how people can be. No I decide, I am much better making all the decisions myself because I knew her and loved her best. I knew my decisions would be made based on love, not greed. After all, I am strong, wise, and experienced, right?! Help!

ICU

Finally it's morning. Did this just happen yesterday? It was a bad dream, right? Reality sets in. No unfortunately, it's very real. OK, I can do this. I get ready to have friends drive me to the hospital. Don't think for one minute, if this happens to you, that you are capable of driving. Even if you have to take a cab, DO!

Mom lies in ICU. She's so helpless; a mere image of the person she was. This can't be happening to me again. My brother was in ICU with tubes everywhere. Unlike my parents and me, Eric's wish was to be kept on life support for two weeks, mainly because of his daughter. He passed the same day they removed the life support.

My dad would have been in ICU too if I hadn't stopped it ahead of time. Let this be a lesson for everyone; if you do not want to be sustained artificially, make sure your loved ones know of your wishes. My dad had suffered a heart attack. They rushed him to the hospital from the nursing home and were going to put him on life support, even though DNR (do not resuscitate) was in his chart. That was his wish. No tubes or life support of any kind. I rushed to the hospital demanding to know why they were going to do this when he was clearly marked DNR. Luckily his doctor fully agreed. He was sent back to the nursing home, on oxygen and medication to make him as comfortable as possible, where he passed peacefully a few days later.

Now here's mom. Her wish the same as dad's. Unfortunately, since she has suffered a stroke her mind isn't working as it normally would. She can't make her wishes clearly known. I talk with her. Assure her it's OK to give up her battle, or it's OK to fight; whatever she wants. She's ready to go. She's confused about what is happening and why she can't function, but knows she doesn't want to continue this way.

I talk to the nurse to see what options we have. Mainly it's a wait and watch for the next 48 hours. The only thing that would sustain her life is a feeding tube since she cannot swallow. The nurse informed me that the doctor had explained this to my mom and she had refused. Now doesn't that tell me something? I say no feeding tube. The nurse explains that if there is no feeding tube then it would be just a matter of days. I say, let's let nature take its course. She is in Higher hands now. I keep praying for her best and highest self. Again I explain she has a living will. No resuscitation, tubes, machines; nothing. Again I am told I need the paperwork now. Once again I have to force my brain into action. I so miss my brain! Please come back to me to help me locate that paperwork!

As we leave the hospital, in the parking lot before reaching the car, I started having a complete breakdown. Everything started spinning. My legs grew weak and shaky. I didn't think they could hold me any longer. Thank God for friends! They got me to the car. How? I don't know. As I sat there, I started shaking, uncontrollably. Me, the strong one, right? I tell myself, breathe, nice deep breaths. My friends are talking to me but I can't make out what they are saying. Listen. Pay attention. They have your best interest at heart. Nothing was making sense. I just knew I had to keep breathing nice deep breaths.

Ok. Better now. Pay attention. What? They want to take me to the emergency room? NOOOOO. Don't worry, I'll snap out of it. "You need to eat", I hear. I respond, "If I do, it will end up on your lap." That is when they knew I had returned to this world somewhat.

When people are under stress, they either overeat, or don't eat. This is normal. Listen to what your body is telling you. Just don't go for an extended abnormal amount of time without eating. This is also why I say you should not drive under these stressful conditions. You might think you can. But like me, you never know when you are going to have a meltdown. Trust me you will. Remember, I was the strong one.

I keep praying and asking for both of our best and highest selves. I learned early in my new "spiritual awakening life" that you can ask for anything from the Angels and from God. This is the best thing I know to do right now for both of us. Ultimately, it is between my mom and her higher self to decide what happens to her. I can only ask for me.

Insight

We arrived at Mom's home. It was much harder walking into her home than I could even begin to imagine. I'm in mom's house, with no mom offering me something to eat, drink, or giving me a treasured trinket she had found. Her smile, her laughter, and her conversation are missing. I know I have been here other times; become impatient to leave or been annoyed for various reasons. I am starting to regret these moments. Will mom ever be able to come back to her home again? Don't think like that. Only concentrate on the good times and on the mission at hand. Focus on that.

 Now, will I be able to find what I need? I am putting the Angels to work as I call upon Them constantly to help me. Not only on an emotional and physical level to find that missing paperwork, but also to help me take actions and make decisions that are for her best and highest self as well as mine. Remember you have to take care of yourself first before you can take care of others.

Just a few months before her stroke, she had shown me where she kept her will and necessary legal paperwork. Did she have a premonition that something was going to happen? I truly believe she had. But did I pay attention to what she had told me? Chances are very slim. Whenever she would try to have these conversations with me, I would put my brain on ignore, into a total state of denial, because this will never happen to my mother, right?

Apparently I must have been listening because not only did I find the necessary paperwork needed now but there were envelopes, neatly labeled and in plain sight of important information I would need for the future. For example, lying on the desk, right above the drawer containing her will was an envelope on which she had written Very Important, underlined it and dated it the beginning of the year. I opened it. It was from her insurance company informing of a policy change which now included long term care. Coincidence? I don't believe in coincidences. I believe everything happens for a reason. Later, as I was cleaning out her things, I found everything was in order, labeled, and easy to find. This wasn't typical behavior for my mom. Trust me she knew something was coming.

Pay attention to these signs with your loved one. Looking back, and now speaking to many people, I truly believe we all have an insight, a sixth sense so to speak, when our time becomes near. Not only had mom shown me where her paperwork was located, but she had made references to friends that she was cleaning house so I wouldn't have so much to do when something happened to her. Everything happens for a reason, right?

The Will

I must now find her will. You have to understand my brain is still not functioning at all. It is just an obstacle, taking up space on top of my neck and shoulders. Did I listen, and do I remember where she told me all the necessary documents were? Thank goodness knowing we would eventually have to put dad in a nursing home due to his Alzheimer's, one very nice person suggested we seek out professional advice from an attorney in regards to all financial aspects, not only for dad's care, but to protect my mother's assets as well. Trust me, for this gentleman to advise us of this was truly a Godsend.

The vast majority of nursing homes or extended care facilities do not inform you of this. In most cases they do not mention financial issues in any way. I advise seeking an attorney who specializes in handling these situations. I also advise having something like a living will or trust completed BEFORE anything happens. I cannot express how important this is to your loved one and to all family members. If we had not sought the help of a professional, dad would have had to pay for all of his care which would have bankrupted my mother. What a shame that would have been. Here were two people that worked all of their lives and saved all of their lives so in their minds they would never have to worry about this exact situation.

If it had not been for this gentleman gently informing us to seek help, there was a good chance not only would mom have lost her money, but her home and car as well. This can and does happen all the time to unknowing but trusting people. Make sure when setting up your will or trust you know exactly the wishes of your loved one and have someone made responsible, given a power of attorney, so those wishes are carried out the way your loved one intended. This may be different from the way the professional people and facilities advise you. After all, they don't know your loved one like you do. Without the proper legal documents, no matter what has been said or discussed, the professionals have to carry out their job to the best of their ability; which can and most likely will become very expensive, but may not be the wish of your loved one.

I find the will. Now remember my brain is not functioning. I search for the part of no resuscitation and anything else I may need. I was able to enlist the help of a friend, Kathy, whose brain was working, and she was able to read upside down! I was correct. No life support of any kind. No machines, tubes, or anything but whatever it takes to make her comfortable. If you or your loved one has a DNR (do not resuscitate), it must get to the medical professionals as soon as possible! It also must go on a colored piece of paper, which is orange in AZ. VERY

Important! In light of this, what can they do to ease her wondering, worrying mind? Her paralysis?

Rest

Back to my house we go. My friends tell me I need to eat and rest. Right! But trust me on this. You really need to take care of yourself when you are in this position. For any of you that have ever flown on an airplane, what do the flight attendants tell you to do in case of an emergency? Yes, take care of yourself first. Put the oxygen mask on YOU first. It will not do your loved ones any good if you are passed out due to lack of oxygen, or in this case, lack of rest, nourishment, and a bundle of nerves. We order pizza which is always my "go to" comfort food. I lie down to sleep. My friends take turns staying with me.

You do NOT want to be alone in these circumstances. I don't care whether it's friends, family, neighbors, or a medical professional. You need anyone whose brain is functioning in case you get that dreaded phone call. Remember I said, even though you think you can, and don't forget I am a very strong independent person, you cannot drive under these conditions. So off to sleep I go. I have had my comfort food and I am in my bed, actually sleeping! When I wake up, this

will all be a dream. Everything will be back to normal.
Guess again!

Wait and Watch

Back to the hospital we go with the necessary paperwork in hand. Frankly, we should have gone to the hospital with the paperwork first but I needed my rest. No change in mom. Is she here or has she gone somewhere else? Hopefully, she is in a peaceful place.

"Now what" I ask. Wait and watch they reply. "For how long?" Only time will tell they say. The next 24 hours will be the most critical. I remind them that mom would never want to live like this. I show them her will. By tomorrow, if she still isn't able to swallow, we will have to put a feeding tube in. "If we don't put the feeding tube in?" Remember, she has already refused it once. Then it will only be a matter of days, since she isn't able to receive proper nourishment. This is all coming from a very caring nurse. It's extremely difficult to speak with the doctor, but it is late at night.

What are her chances? What can I expect next? Even with all of my medical background, I have no idea what to expect, or even what questions to ask. The nurse tries to reassure me that since this happened in a casino where she received immediate medical care and most importantly oxygen within minutes, that she has a good chance at survival.

I ask myself, for what? Her life to end, or for the life to be sucked out of her? I don't want that to happen, but even more significant, she wouldn't. If I had been thinking clearly, I would have known that neither the nurse nor anyone else could tell me what to expect. It is all up to mom and a Higher authority. Let's just wait and watch. Don't get mad, or frustrated, I tell myself. She is in good hands. Let's just wait and watch.

24 Hours Later

I go back the next day with my friend Judy and she seems a little better. What's this? A feeding tube is in her nose! Why? The doctor talked her into it. But she refused yesterday. I have her paperwork, her will, stating she wants no machines, tubes, nothing! Now the doctor talks her into it! I demand to see the doctor. I don't care if it is Sunday morning. This is my mother!

The doctor informs me that without the feeding tube, due to her size (little), age (old), she would only last a few days at best. Isn't that her wish? Isn't that what is in her will? Why wasn't I informed? I'm told it wasn't my decision to make. Really? Margaret's the one who suffered brain damage with the stroke. Yet, you believe she can think straight? Don't think so. What is it? You want more money? I know the medical professionals have to do their job especially in this law suit happy world. But I thought that I would have at least been consulted on this matter.

To tell the truth though, I'm glad I didn't have to make that decision. I know no matter what the outcome, I would have questioned my choice. So emotionally I'm better off letting the professionals take over on this one. Like I really had a choice.

The doctor explains to me the various scenarios that might happen. I understand every case is different, but all I'm asking for is some direction, some expectation. Most importantly what can I do? He gives me all the medical explanations. Thank goodness I comprehend. If you are fortunate enough to understand medical terms, procedures, etc., good for you. If not, take someone along who does understand, or at least have someone by your side to ask questions. Keep asking until you do understand even if it frustrates or angers the medical staff.

Bottom line, the best thing for mom at this time is to keep talking to her, reassuring her. Having friends come over to give her comfort. No problem, I'm on it! I sit with her for hours talking with her as I would normally do, stroking her hand, and telling her how much I love her. I let her know I am doing everything I can to help her including talking with the Angels and God.

My friends are also there reassuring her and letting her know they are taking care of me. In typical mother style she is still more worried about my well-being than she is her own. I truly believe the main reason she, and so many others like her, stay around so long is that not only do they have to make their peace with their God or Higher Power, but they also are worried about their loved ones. What will happen to them if I die?

I was astounded when the nurse talked to me about how so many people lie in these beds all alone. She was so happy about how many visitors mom had even though it was just me and five of my dear friends. Wouldn't that just be terrible to go through something like this all alone?

Progress

Days go by. She is getting better; at least becoming more aware, but is still just a mere skeleton of herself. She doesn't seem to be quite so scared, or is that just an act? The medical personnel are very nice. They have scans, blood work, x-rays, and tests ordered every day. Is all this really necessary? What can change in a day? I am not consulted or advised. They just do their thing.

Within a week she is moved to a regular room. "Ok now what?" I ask. She will be here for about two weeks. If she continues to improve, she will go to rehab. "Where is that and what do they do?" Even with 20 plus years in the medical field, brother died of AIDS, father in nursing home with Alzheimer's, I had no clue as to what really goes on in rehab. I learned really quickly, if I wanted answers, ask questions. And ask a lot! They do not volunteer information.

I found out in rehab they will teach her many things that just a week ago she took for granted. They will work with her to help her adjust to her paralysis by re-teaching her how to walk, talk, think, and use her arm. But will she be able to go home? Will she be able to walk, use her arm, and control her bodily functions? This was the part she felt the most ashamed about. Not having control over her bodily functions. Not so much the urine aspect, but the bowels.

"Will she be able to eat?" Probably not, they reply. "Great! How long does she need to have that tube down her nose?" Two to three weeks at the most since that is the longest the human body can tolerate, I'm told. Longer and the body would start to reject it. If it was me, I would have rejected it from the start. But not Margaret, boy did she prove them wrong!

Rehab

After about a total of two weeks in the hospital, I go to visit one afternoon and they are packing her things. "What's this?" I ask. We are moving her to rehab. "Really? Doesn't anyone call in to inform you of anything anymore? Where is rehab?" You can follow us. Thank goodness I was there when I was and was able to follow.

Not that it did me any good. The hospital she was in is huge. We go through underground tunnels for quite some time and then we are in a whole different building. How we got there and how do I get back to my car was for me to figure out later. After asking, I did have someone show me around the rehab facility. It seems nice enough, clean enough. What I didn't like was that I was given no choice in the matter. What if I didn't like it here? More importantly, what if mom didn't? I have to trust and rely on the professionals. It would have been nice to have someone explain things to me before they happened. Again, it goes back to what I have said before, ASK!

They show me a board that has her schedules, such as baths and different therapy times. I ask what each therapy is for and what is done. I know they are professionals. I have to trust and rely on them to make the correct choices for her, but it is still scary. As I walk through the facility, many of the patients are frightening to me. They can't sit up, breathe on their own, talk, or anything. Bless their hearts, I know this is not their fault, but is this how mom will end up in rehab? I just have to keep trusting and believing in the best for her. Angels please help!

Many questions go through my brain. Yes my brain is starting to function again. I say that very liberally, considering it went into hiding for a while! How long will all of this take? What will be her condition in the end? I ask if there is anyone who can explain to me in detail and hopefully in a way that I can understand, what happens next. I am informed they have counselors who can help me with my questions and expectations. I am encouraged to join mom for all of her therapies. Thank goodness, I do not have a "real" job, or a family at home I need to take care of. Just another illustration of the good and the bad of being all by yourself.

I tried calling the counselor a few times, but to no avail. I did attend many of mom's therapy sessions. I must say, the therapists were extremely professional, nice and informative. I watched, to my amazement, her continual improvement. Her speech was getting better and she was able to function with her impairment better. Even her mind seemed a little better although definitely not totally back to normal.

Mom tells me she has visions of "people" visiting her room. Everyone from TV personalities, (the ones she mentioned were actually people she had met), to Angels, and deceased loved ones. I ask myself, what this all means. I am a psychic/medium. I have helped people cross over and I help people in this life see their deceased loved ones and deliver comforting messages. I see Angels and deliver their messages to my clients. This is different. I am too close to my mother. I cannot figure out, is she getting ready to cross over, or is she in for the battle of a life time?

The Hunt

After about two weeks in rehab with continual improvement, the elusive counselor appears on a late Friday afternoon. He informs me that mom has to be moved to a nursing home. What? Why? I'm told they need the room, but later find it's more of an insurance issue. What I learned is that over the course of mom's incapacitation, everything was dictated by the insurance company and the professional's interpretation of what the insurance company was going to permit. Now isn't that a shame? Trust me mom had the best of the best insurance. Do you? And if you don't, what would happen to you?

So I ask, "How do I go about finding her a nursing home?" I'm handed a book. "What do I do with this?" Here's a list. "Can you recommend a place?" Legally, I know he cannot but he does circle several that are close to where I live that he has heard were good.

Home I go to make calls on a late Friday afternoon. Oh did I tell you, she has to be out of there by the following Tuesday? Good luck trying to reach someone on a Friday afternoon. I leave messages at several facilities but receive no return calls over the weekend. Apparently the people you need to consult with don't work on weekends.

On Monday I go to the VA where we had placed my dad. He had lived so well there, I was hoping it would work for mom. As I toured the facility again, (NOOO! This can't be happening again, can it!?) I decided it was perfect for dad being a WWII vet, but since mom was not in the war it wouldn't be for her. Next I went to visit the only other facility that returned my call, out of about eight I tried.

The lady I met with was very nice and caring. The facility was clean, and as an added bonus, it was close to my house. It also provided the three therapies she would need in order to improve. Not all nursing homes provide therapy. If your loved one needs therapy, ask ahead of time. Inspect the therapy rooms and talk with the therapists. You have the right. Can you tell my brain was getting stronger? Oh how I had missed it! If they do not let you see the rooms where they stay, sleep, eat, bathe, and take therapy, or whatever it is you feel the need to examine, leave! No, run! Imagine how they will care for your loved one if they are not showing you what you want to see, or potentially hiding things from you.

Also very important, ASK questions. Talk to other patients, family members, nurses, aides, and even the cleaning crew. This is your loved one being cared for. Make sure you are comfortable with everything. Of course there will be some things you might not like.

Just like buying a house or car, nothing is ever 100% perfect. But is it something you can live with? Also, from the very beginning, ask about insurance. Don't let them evade this issue or cover it up, which is something they do very well. TRUST ME! If I hadn't been well informed by the gentleman at the VA facility where my dad stayed, I would have been in the dark once again.

Seek professional help. If you have a chance, make this one of the very first things you do when something happens to your loved one. Then when you are given two days to move them, you are informed and can ask and make intelligent choices.

Ask friends, family, or neighbors for the name(s) of attorneys you can consult. Many attorneys will provide an initial consultation for approximately one hour for free. Some want to charge you $200-$500. It all depends on your financial position. My opinion, why pay for something if you are not going to use it? Mind you, these consultations are only to give advice. Obtain several professional opinions. Take someone with you either a family member or friend. You are going through a very stressful time. You may not be able to understand or remember everything an attorney tells you if you are alone. So bring someone for backup.

Here are some of the questions I asked. Is this covered under her insurance? Will there be any out of pocket expenses she is required to pay? Will I be informed ahead of time of any required expenses? How long will she be here? What can I expect now and in the future? Will she be assigned a doctor, or do I have to get one?

In this facility, they assigned Margaret one of their doctors. Since she had the best of the best insurance, all expenses would be covered as long as she continued to improve. That was the million dollar phrase! "What if she didn't continue to improve?" Then the insurance would quit paying and all expenses would have to come out of her pocket, which trust me, wasn't that deep. "How much is it?" $5500 a month I was told. You're kidding, right? Ok. I'll deal with that later.

The Move

I inform rehab that I had found a nursing home for her. I was told she couldn't be moved. She has a bladder infection, which has to be treated before she can be moved. "You were going to tell me about this, when? How long will she need to stay here?" I have to contact the nursing home and tell them she won't be coming as planned. A scary thought runs through my mind. What if the nursing home fills up? This can and does happen so make sure you have a backup plan. Of course rehab can't tell me how much longer she will be there. That's right, wait and watch.

It is now the evening of Friday, July 3rd. I receive a phone call that they are moving her tonight. "Can't you wait until the morning? This will confuse her even more." They need the bed. Good news is they handle all the transportation arrangements. "Can I at least receive a phone call when she has been transported?" They agree and I receive the call at 10:00 p.m. How they can move someone who is 87 years old at that time of night is way beyond me. Again I have no say. I thought I told you, I lost my brain, not my voice. I cannot go visit because it is after hours. Now I'm wracked with worry about how mom will adjust. Well there goes what little brain I had recovered.

I cannot stress enough here how many times I have asked for help from friends and from the Angels and God. I am not used to asking for human help, only help from the Higher side. I really don't know how I would have survived even at this point without all of them helping me. Not even a month has transpired at this point and I have had several melt downs. It's nerve racking never knowing what the future will bring, or even getting just a little clue. After all, we're dealing with my mother's life here. I have no control or say in any of the decision making except for what facility to move her into. Little did I know that this was just barely the beginning of what I would be asked to handle.

The Nursing Home

It is now the morning of July 4th. I am given her room number by the receptionist. I go to her room but she's not there! I had made prior arrangements that she have a bed by the window, overlooking a courtyard. She loved the outdoors. Frantically I go to all the surrounding rooms in search of mom. She is nowhere to be found. Did something happen? My mind is a blur. I'm in panic mode; unable to find anyone to assist me. Finally I find a nurse dispensing medication. She seemed agitated at my interruption. Do you think I really care? This is my mother! I ask politely if she knew where my mom was. Begrudgingly, she replied she had no idea and continued with her work. I pick up her clipboard, slamming it down, repeating again, where is my MOTHER!

Now I have her full attention. I don't care if she thinks I'm crazy. Why do I have to go to these extremes? If they had made the arrangements we previously had agreed upon this wouldn't be happening. It is not my nature to be mean. Twice now in less than a month I have picked up a medical professional's clipboard and slammed it down to receive answers to my questions. And both times it was simply where in the world is my mother!!

It has only been three weeks since her stroke. I have already lost 10 lbs. I'm not able to eat. When I try, even just some yogurt, my hand shakes so bad I can't even hold the spoon. It is pure hell never knowing what the next day of trauma is going to bring. Will I receive the "dreaded phone call"? Does she have to be moved again with no help or notice? Will she have another stroke?

I have so many unanswered questions. But as a mother protects their child, it is now role reversal. I will do anything to protect the woman who brought me into this world! The nurse finds out I was given the wrong room number. Really? Duh! I go into a room which was not the one we had made arrangements for. She is lying in the bed facing the hallway. Mom's very disoriented, confused, and scared. Didn't I tell you this would happen? I spend most of the day with her, trying to comfort and reassure. Is she listening? Does she even comprehend?

Finally, I go home to get some much needed rest. I return that evening, to see her just lying there, but not really there. She tells me about the Angels she is seeing, my deceased father and brother, her deceased father and mother. Since I am a psychic dealing in Angel readings, and a medium dealing with communicating with deceased loved ones, I encourage her to tell me what she is seeing and hearing. I am sensing that her time is drawing near.

She seems very peaceful, almost wishful. Wouldn't you if you had Angels and your deceased loved ones all around you?

First thing Monday morning I am at the administrative office finding out why she was not placed in the agreed upon room and where were her clothes? Yes, that's right. I had taken some of her clothes to rehab. They want them to be in as natural a surrounding as possible, in their own clothes as opposed to the hospital gowns. Not thinking, I took some of her favorite clothes. Mom was a flashy dresser. Apparently the clothes did not make the move with mom. When do these battles quit?

You might be saying to yourself, that I just had a bad experience. This doesn't happen all the time. Think again. Actually, after talking with many people, my experiences are NOTHING compared to what others have gone through. But remember I am strong, and most of all determined!

The nursing home makes arrangements to have her moved to the original room, like there was any doubt. I'm introduced to the head housekeeper who was in search of her clothes. Since they were not found, the blame was shifted back to the hospital/rehab. Yes I did call them. No they did not have her clothes. And believe it or not the clothes were never found. Fortunately I was instructed to send an itemized statement of her clothes including the value and I was reimbursed. But that was cold comfort when compared with the fact that mom had lost some of her favorite things.

I am now introduced to her nurses, aides, and therapists. Once again I am encouraged to attend therapies with her. I keep asking myself, how can people do this when they have a "real" job, family, live out of state, or have a spouse? How do their spouses handle this; especially the elderly ones, the couples who have been married 40, 50, 60, years? Those spouses could now be in their 80's, 90's. Maybe they too are in bad health and their primary caretaker has now become the patient. And I think my problems are extreme!

This is probably what keeps me somewhat sane. I think about these people. I pray for these people. I see them all the time at the nursing home. Then I tell myself, it could be worse for me. What if my dad was still alive and living at home, by himself now with Alzheimer's? Even worse, what if my brother was still alive, living in Kansas and I receive the "dreaded phone call" better come quick? Not much time left. How would I manage?

No matter how bad you think it is for you at the present moment, it could always be worse. I truly believe, these thoughts, my protective instincts, and let's not forget about my belief in God and Angels, is what kept my sanity, such as it was, intact. Trust me I am using the word sanity extremely liberally!

Progress

I am seeing a significant improvement in her condition. Her speech is improving and her thinking is clearer. Even her sense of humor is coming back. Is she going to pull through this? Was it just a month ago, I was given a 40% survival rate? Mom's still not eating much, which has the caretakers quite concerned. She is just a little person anyway, but how could you eat with a tube down your nose? Wasn't that supposed to be removed within two weeks and it now is going on six weeks? I tried to talk with the doctor about this but unless you are physically there in person when the doctor is making his rounds, there is not much chance of talking with him. I ask how I can meet with him. Address questions? Communicate? I'm informed about the time and day he is there. So I wait.

Finally we meet. Very nice caring overall good guy! Great! We have a long talk. Yes she is improving. Her constant pain in her paralyzed side, (isn't that strange they have pain in their paralyzed side? You would think it would be numb), is normal. It probably will never go away.

The doctor informs me we have to remove the feeding tube. You think? He wants to take her to the hospital to place a feeding tube in her stomach which requires surgery. No more I say. She has been through enough. Remember, she is DNR - do not resuscitate. He thoroughly agreed, but also said without a feeding tube she would probably only last a few days, a week at the most. We agreed to allow her to make that decision. Whew, another load off of me.

Mom agreed with us. She doesn't want to go through anymore. We are all in agreement to allow nature to take its course. The doctor said he would cancel all of her therapies and have hospice come in. There's that word, hospice. Do you really know what hospice is or does? I thought hospice was only brought in when there is only a very short time left on this physical plane. As you will later learn, that is not necessarily the case.

Mom and I look at each other, not sure we are on the same page with his recommendation. Mom and I decided to allow the therapies and no hospice for one week to see what happens. The doctor agrees. Her feeding tube is pulled on a Friday. By Monday, she went from eating mush food to solids! No, this lady was not giving up without a fight! Meanwhile, I'm at home for those three days waiting for that call telling me my mother is gone. Evaluating, have I made the right decision? Then assuring myself it wasn't my decision, it was Margaret's.

Visits from the Other Side

Progress is being made daily. She goes to a small dining area to have aides help her with eating. She cannot be left alone to eat since her throat is still not working properly, which could cause her to choke to death. Also there is interaction with three other patients. Mom really loves her time here, probably due to the extra attention. After several weeks of being in the smaller dining area, they let us know she will be transferred to a bigger dining area. This truly confuses and scares her! It's a much bigger room. There are more patients. Many people are in various stages of physical, as well as mental distress. Most can't even sit up on their own, let alone talk. Not as much personal attention. Did they explain why she had to be moved? I wonder how much are they really telling to their patients? How much are the patients capable of understanding? How much do I comprehend? Where is there a counselor or a guidance person to help eliminate the confusion, the fears?

I know I have my own fears and confusion. But my brain isn't damaged. Or is it? I can only imagine what fears, confusion, frustrations, and demons my mom is battling. Oh how I would like to be in her head so I could help her. Her frustrations, not only of being physically handicapped, but the mental anxiety, the humiliation of having no control over bodily organs, primarily, her bladder and bowels. She is now reduced to having to rely on people, much like a new born baby does. I can't even begin to understand her exasperation at not being able to communicate, or even have her thoughts process properly. Let's see. Was it just two months ago she was in a casino, winning over $200 in 20 minutes? Seems like an eternity ago.

Not that this isn't enough, but she is continuously seeing dead people. Again my father, brother, her father, mom, sister, Angels and Spirit Guides are appearing. Is her time drawing nearer? She tells me she wants to go just like her mother. I ask how her mom passed. Margaret tells me her mother came to help her to the white light. Being spiritually gifted, I help her by giving her an understanding of the other side. I help her see and feel the white light; the love, comfort, and peace; the overall well-being. Does she understand? Does it scare or comfort her? Is she mentally still here on this earth plane, or has her spirit connected into the spiritual realm?

One day mom tells me that an old neighbor friend, Tiny, from Ohio came in for a visit. She went into great detail how Tiny had come all the way to visit her and sat on the chair right next to her bed. I explained, knowing very well this hadn't happened, that it was highly doubtful since this lady had been extremely ill as well. You have to be very careful what you say and how you say it, so as to not confuse them further causing more anxiety. I learned this extremely well with my father's Alzheimer's. She insisted that it did happen. Two days later I received a phone call from one of mom's close neighbor friends inquiring about mom's condition. After chatting for a bit she informed me, without knowing about mom's "visit" that Tiny had just passed recently. Was this a coincidence? I don't believe in coincidences!

Back to Me

Meanwhile, here I am back at home trying to maintain my sanity. After all, if I lose it who will watch over mom? Many people keep gently telling me to get on with my life, including her doctor. What life? Again, I say thank God I don't have a real job, or family to take care of. Is this a curse or blessing? Maybe it would be better if I had something other than my mom to focus on. But knowing me, that wouldn't work either. I would constantly be asking myself if I should be with her. What else could I, or should I be doing? It doesn't matter because this is my life. This is the hand I have been dealt, (yes I do love to play cards), so this is how I have to play the game. Thank goodness for my friends, allowing me to call at all times of the day or night. I sleep, drink, watch TV, and read. Anything I can do to maintain and take my mind away from the matters at hand.

On the advice of friends and the medical professionals, mainly her doctor that I truly believe in, I am no longer visiting her every day. My brain is slowly coming back to me. Boy, how I have so missed my brain. Not to be confused with fully functioning, but I am starting to think and planning for the future, whatever that might bring. What about all the paperwork, banking, automatic deposits, automatic withdrawals, and all of these bills that are piling up? Is the insurance paying them, or is she responsible? What about her personal items and her home? I can't handle all of this yet can I? You must, the little voice in my head tells me.

Her neighbors are a blessing. They watch after her home for me. They watch out after me, for me. They call me and visit her on a regular basis. They allow me to visit them to talk and cry but mainly to listen and have a shoulder to lean on. Her one neighbor brings up the one question I have been avoiding like the plague - what are you going to do with her home?

Mom lived in a mobile home park. Very nice. Home is paid for. The only problem, rent was running over $600 a month. What if I need that money somewhere in the future for her care? Will she fully recover and want to come home, or will she pass tomorrow?

Blessedly, her neighbor and friend sit me down and have a long talk with me. See her brain is working. She explains even if mom does progress to a point where she no longer requires the nursing home, she will always need professional care. But what she said to me that really struck a chord was that Margaret would never be able to take care of the yard again, nor sit out on her porch without assistance. And that would cause mom great pain. It would really be for the best to sell her home.

Great! Now what does that bring? Do you know how much "stuff" she has in her home? We are about to find out! I know, not only from my personal experiences, but also with others, people who survived the depression never throw anything away. Most are not pack rats, they just remember a time in their life when there was nothing. Once again, I put on my big girl pants to see what lies before me.

Paperwork

I had been to her house many times since her stroke but it was never the same. I couldn't stay there for long. Too many memories and too many unanswered questions would go through my head. I had only been there to get essentials; her clothes, toiletries, paperwork. Being of sound mind all of her life, I had never handled any of her paperwork such as banking, insurance, utilities, etc. I didn't even know where to look for all of this. Does any of this sound familiar to you?

I knew she had closed one bank account, and had opened several others. Hopefully they were all at the same bank. We had never discussed this in full detail. Please let that be a lesson to all of you out there. Always have someone know where important papers are kept, no matter what your age or condition. Another word to the wise, try to have at least one friend at the bank or financial institution you do business with. In times such as these, you cannot think straight. You do need a friend on your side to help guide you, someone that is there for you, not the corporation they work for. They can assist you with your best interest at heart, and still not get into trouble with their company.

It was my good fortune that mom and I had made friends with several people at the bank. One such person, advised me almost from the start to shut off her phone and cable service. Why pay for that? It can always be turned back on. You can have the phone number forwarded to any number you choose.

I start going through her personal paperwork. It feels so strange. Even though this is my mother, I feel I am invading her privacy. I put these thoughts and feelings to rest. It has to be done. It is for her best interest. I get a handle on automatic withdrawals and deposits. Bless her heart. She is a very organized and detail minded person. It wasn't hard to find these essential items, even though they were scattered throughout her home; in cabinets, dressers, nightstands, desk drawers, under the bed, and in closets. Thank goodness her home is small. Everything was labeled and in perfect order.

I find out later she had made comments to several friends that she was putting everything in order and getting rid of a bunch of things so my job wouldn't be so hard to do when the time comes. See, I told you, no matter our age, we all have a feeling when our time draws near. Even though everything was well organized, I still found paid bills, receipts, and paperwork of all sorts that she had kept for years. I am not talking one or two or even seven years. I found things dated as much as 20 years ago! People, get rid of it! Unless it is very personal to you, i.e. birth certificate, marriage license, tax paperwork, letters, etc. please dispose of it! Not only is it terribly time consuming for the person(s) having to go through all of this, but it is also a fire hazard.

Now that I have all the paperwork, what does it all mean? My first instinct is to go to an attorney to receive legal counsel to help me sort through all of this. Knowing from my Dad's experience, if she had to go to a place which would be self-pay her money would run out in a matter of months. Then what? I feel it is such a shame, my parents, born in 1920's lived through WWII, of which my father served in the army, the depression, worked hard all of their lives, saved, provided for their family, did everything they were taught and learned to do, finding now, there is no financial help for them. Here is my mother, receiving excellent benefits, since my father was a state employee, now in a position where she could lose everything and have no care provided for her. Is this why we work hard and save, just to be left stranded on the streets when we need help?

Legal Counsel

I was referred to an attorney, whom, when I called wanted $250 just for a 1 hour consultation. I knew after going through a divorce, this was common. I also knew I was not going to receive help other than just advice, but was hoping I could take that information and run with it. Understand, I felt the need to be proactive in the event her insurance was taken away.

I did discover a few avenues that were available to her. One, she was entitled to financial aid through the VA. It doesn't matter that she did not serve. My dad was a vet, thus entitling the spouse for benefits once the insurance stopped. That is the good news. The bad news is it can take 6-9 months to receive that help. And that is only if the paperwork you submit the first time is completely correct. If not, they will send it all back to you. Then you have to discover the error, correct, and then resubmit. Really, why does this have to be so difficult? My dad served his country. He did his fair share. This is how they repay him?

I also learned of several other avenues we could take, but in order to pursue them the attorney wanted $4,000 to start and went up from there. How much further up I'm asking myself. Do I allow the attorney to explore these avenues, having no guarantees they will even work for mom? Or do I hold onto the money and pray for the best?

Thank God for friends! A very good friend of mine had a friend, who was in a similar situation with her mother. She sought legal counsel as well, and referred me to her attorney which she assured me she completely liked, but more importantly trusted. And no consultation fee! Imagine. Sign me up. I knew instantly when I met this attorney that he was the one for me. Not only was he extremely nice, knowledgeable, helpful, and reasonable, but he truly seemed genuine, caring, understanding, and passionate.

I really needed someone that was on my side for a change. I knew I wasn't his first client to go through this, and I wouldn't be his last. Trust me, it is difficult enough to handle all aspects of making sure my mother is being provided for in the best way possible, but to go it alone is even harder. The only good part about being by yourself is you don't have anyone else to fight or question your every intention.

I thank God every day for being there for me, and my high spiritual beliefs. Thank goodness I have learned over the years to trust my heart, gut, and listening to those little voices in my head. This attorney was right for me! Now I finally had someone helping me I felt I could trust. At least on the financial part and hopefully in the battles that I knew were lying ahead of me! How many more battles are there to be fought? Won?

Back at the Ranch
(Nursing Home)

Mom continues to eat, now without help. She can eat in her room or the dining room. It's her choice. Friends and I would take turns to be with her at dinner time. I had to stop going every day. Mentally and physically, I just couldn't take it anymore. Even her doctor tells me to get back to my life. Right! This is my life. This IS my mother, who I have to take care of and watch over. Trust me, not an easy decision to make. The guilt always sets in. But as I tell my clients, how can you take care of others, if you don't first take care of you? Thank God for friends! Phyllis, Kathy, Lorraine, Judy, Joe, Jeanne, mom's neighbors all take turns visiting and staying with her. This really helped. I know they are doing this for mom because they love her, but they love me as well.

She has now been in this nursing home about six weeks. It's been a full two months after her stoke, when the doctor gave me less than a 40% survival rate. Seems like a life time ago! She keeps steadily improving. Guess she's not ready to give up yet, at least not without a fight!

I receive a phone call late in the afternoon from someone at the nursing home whom I have never met. Why do they always wait until late in the day to call? Again I ask what if I had a real job. This person informs me I have three days to move my mother. I wondered who this person was, since my mom and I had gotten to know just about everyone involved with her care. So who is this unknown stranger telling me I have to move mom and why?

I'm told it's because the insurance will no longer pay for her care because she is not continuing to improve. Who said she is not improving? I had just spoken with the doctor and he was amazed at her improvement. I am informed it came from a therapist. Trust me when this happens, and it does on a very frequent basis to everyone, not just us, they expect you to roll over and take it. They don't know who they are messing with. I could totally understand if she wasn't making progress, but she was.

I go down there with guns blazing, so to speak. I meet with the person with the power to be. She says that mom is not eating. She only weighs 100 lbs. That's how much she weighed when she had her stroke. Her response, she's not eating enough. Mom never did. She was also informed by the therapist that mom is not improving.

I go marching to therapy. Last week I was told mom was improving more than anyone thought would be possible. She has learned how to use her good side to help her paralyzed one. She is able to maneuver herself to the side of the bed and, to get into a wheelchair that she can control by herself. Now they're saying there's no improvement? What part of this therapy indicates she is not improving? Just in as little a time as one month ago, she was not able to do any of this!

Remember when the doctor pulled her feeding tube and wanted to bring in hospice because he gave her about 2-3 days to live at best? She not only is eating on her own but able to move on her own. Please explain to me, where you see this as no improvement? I might as well have been talking to a brick wall. Trust me, that wall would have had more answers than these people.

I wait until late afternoon for her doctor to arrive. After a lengthy discussion, he too is clueless but not surprised. He said, this is very common and they do this all the time. He informs me I can protest this. Now how am I to know that I have the right to protest? Trust me there are NO nursing home 101 classes. You learn by trial and error. He instructs me to write a letter explaining I am protesting this dismissal including the reasons why. He also said he would sign it and help me fight it. When he fights a dismissal, he wins about 90% of the time. Could I possibly have another professional on my side? Yea! But I wonder, what happens the other 10% of the time?

I can't let that bother or worry me now. At this point I have nothing to lose, except to keep her here and pay close to $200 a day, yes $200 a DAY! People had asked why I didn't move mom in with me. I was not physically or emotionally able to have her stay with me 24 hour a day times 7 days a week. These people were able to give free advice over the phone without visiting me or mom in person to truly understand either one of our physical or emotional conditions.

I truly was grateful to have a professional take time to talk with me, educate me, and really care. Again, I ask myself, what do people do when they have their spouse in there and they are 80 or 90 some years young. Or maybe they themselves are not in good health. What do these people do? Do they have the fight in them that I do? Or do they just trust and believe in the system? Don't!

The Guidance and Help

Several days go by with no phone call. What does this mean? Do I have to move her or not, and if I do, where? How much? Is no news good news, or will I get a call to move her today? As I am walking down the street for my daily walk, (Yes exercise is the best medicine and a great stress reliever, and for me it gives me a chance to connect with the Angels. Without my Angels, God, and my belief system in place, I would have been in a worse institution than mom was in!), my neighbor stops to inquire about mom. She had to put her dad in a home early that year, so was familiar with some of what I was going through. I informed her of what was happening. Her response to me was, why don't you use a head hunter? A what? Her sister had gone online and found out there were people who will help you find the perfect home for your loved one. They are nick named "head hunters". They absolutely loved their gal and found their father the perfect home.

"What does that cost?" Nothing! The Head Hunter receives her money from the home she places them in. All you have to do is tell her what you are looking for, price range, area, and those kinds of things. She does her homework and then will drive you around, much like a realtor, to find a home you feel will be a perfect match. My neighbor explained they really liked this person not only because she was very knowledgeable, but also because she truly cares.

My neighbor confides in me that this particular head hunter went through the same thing when her husband was diagnosed at an early age with a terminal disease. She too had to place him in a home and had to keep moving him because she didn't like the care he was being given. Now she wants to help others so they don't have to go through the pain that she went through. (Much like this book, right?) Wow I think to myself. What a concept. Does this mean I can have another professional on my side?

I give her a call. She's fantastic! She totally understands the situation and even gave me helpful advice on how to handle the nursing home situation. I explain, I don't know when I will have to move mom, but I want to be proactive. This has already happened to us twice, I want to be ready if and when, knowing darn good and well, it would happen in the future. Maybe not today or tomorrow, but I knew it would happen. Why can't there be a better consistent system in place. Is this how to treat our elderly? Do you think they want to be in this kind of physical condition? I can't speak for all the elderly, but I know my mother definitely wouldn't want this!

The Hunt Resumed

My head hunter, Becky, is a dream come true. Another Angel sent from God! Thank you! We meet. I explain what I feel would be a good fit for mom. Since mom and I both disliked hospitals, I didn't want her to be in a home that looked, felt and smelled like a hospital. I also didn't want anything too large. I wanted loving caring people, close to where I lived, and of course inexpensive! Since this was her profession she knew most of the homes all over the valley. This is Phoenix, city of retirees, so there are many to choose from.

She does her research based on my criteria and off we go. Before we get to each home, Becky explains its "personality"; the good, bad and ugly. The places we looked at were all private homes with only 6-12 patients per home. The caretakers were amazing; extremely nice, genuine, and most important, caring people. How they do what they do, I have no idea, but bless them. The homes were amazing. It would be like walking into your own home, just with people that needed care. There were no smells, just clean, updated, and nice! I found one I felt would be a perfect match but had two backups just in case mom didn't have to move for a while and my first choice became full. I'm learning! As you will later read, this is very important. Anything you do, always have a backup plan.

Not only did she find me the perfect home, but informed me my mother was entitled to financial aid through the VA since my dad was a vet. Gee where I have I heard this before. Oh yes. From someone who charged me $250! Becky had the perfect person for me to meet who would handle all the paperwork and get it all done in three months or less at no charge. I also find out, once everything becomes approved, it is retroactive. You're kidding, another person on my side. Wow they are lining up! But I continue to caution myself, don't get too excited. You never know when or what other bomb might drop.

Back to the Fight

Back to the nursing home I go. About a week has transpired. I have heard nothing. Are they keeping her, or booting her? I talk to the Director. It's no surprise to me anymore, no one knows anything. What do I do, continue to wait until I get that phone call late in the day? Will mom be here forever, or will she have to be moved tomorrow?

I'm counseled not to worry until I hear from her. Easy for her to say! "If you find out I have to move mom, can I be given some kind of notice so I can let these homes I found know in advance?" The Director can't guarantee that will happen. Now you might be asking at this point, why I didn't just move her. There were a few reasons.

Money was one main issue. These homes are not inexpensive. They can range anywhere from $1500 a month up to $10,000, which is not covered under Medicare or any other insurance, other than the financial aid through the VA. The current nursing home was covered 100% by her insurance. My mother was not wealthy. She lived on social security and a small retirement fund, plus I was still paying rent on her mobile home (just in case), which was averaging now around $650 a month since electric was included and it was summer time in Phoenix, Az.

I did check on getting her around the clock nursing care in the event she was able to move back to her home. These agencies charge an average of $20 per hour. That would be 24 hours a day times 7 days per week times 52 weeks per year. Do the math, it's expensive. In addition, with the nursing home she was in, she could continue with all of her therapies. Once again, we were in a wait and watch situation, never knowing what the next day would bring.

Now I understand this is life, but she is now living under a controlled environment, with professional people. Again I ask, where are the counselors or guidance people to keep you informed, or at least act like they want you prepared for all situations? Why do I have to go to bed every night with so many unanswered questions and a huge knot in my belly? No wonder I can't eat.

Selling

Mom's very loving neighbors finally talked me into putting her mobile home up for sale. She would never be able to live there again unless she made a full recovery, which was highly unlikely. One of her best friends said it would break mom's heart not to be able to go outside to do the yard work she loved or to visit with her friends. This broke my heart but I saw the wisdom in what they were saying.

There were many homes for sale in her park with none of them selling. The few that were selling, were taking many months, if not a year or longer to sell. Remember this is 2009 in Phoenix, a city that was hit hard in the real estate market. Now in addition to all of the other unknowns I am dealing with, I have to make arrangements to sell the home that she has lived in for more than 20 years and dispose of her personal belongings, many that have been with her a whole lifetime. Is this ever going to end?

I invited many friends over to take whatever they wanted. I had no room. Luckily for me, they came to work, thank God! I was an emotional wreck. I could not think. Normally I am usually in charge. Every time someone asked me a question I looked at them with a blank stare or broke down crying, which is not like me.

I was invading someone's privacy. Even though it was my mother's it was still extremely difficult to handle. What should I take? What stays? Who wants what? What do I do with the "leftovers"? How can I part with things that have been in my parent's possession for more than 50 years? I know these are only materialistic things, but they are sentimental. Will I ever see them again? Will they disappear out of my life like my brother, father, and probably soon my mother? How can I go on? Thank God, my friends are very protective. They wrap, pack, ask if they could have..., told me to keep..., but I was fully aware they were more concerned about me, than the "things", because all I could do is sit in my mother's chair and sob.

We all went back the following week to finish as much as we could. Mentally I was in a better condition to do this. I was over the initial "shock". Now much has been removed. Friends took what they wanted, or brought to my house what they felt I shouldn't part with at this time. But you have to understand, my parents grew up in the great depression so they didn't part with anything. There was still much more to do in order to have the house show well for potential buyers. It just amazed me how someone's valuable "stuff" can become "junk," overnight. If mom had knowledge of this, I'm sure it would have caused her to pass more quickly than the results of the stroke.

Blessedly, a friend of mine was able to put me in contact with a shelter that helped all types of people in needy situations. They would come over and take anything. Even bag or box it for you and haul it off to dispense to those needy people. I had such a good feeling about this group of volunteers who came to get mom's valuables. Before they even started, they asked what situation had happened to cause these circumstances. I explained everything. We went into mom's bedroom, joined hands, and unknown to me, the one gentleman was a minster who said a very extensive prayer, not only for mom, but included me as well. A very generous, and loving act of kindness. I knew I had made the right choice.

Continuance

Mom proceeds to improve over the next weeks. However, she continues to see "dead" people now on a daily basis. She starts repeating conversations she is having with, not only my deceased father and brother, but also with her deceased, father, mother, sisters, and brothers-in-law. Again she tells me she wants to go just the way her mother did. Being psychic and a medium I know what this all means, but feel helpless.

I work with her to see the light, the Angels, God; anything to give her peace, comfort, and reassurance. But as I have learned in these past two years, it is not about us, it's about the agreement individuals made with their higher being before they arrived on this earth plane. **They** are the ones who have to make it right before they can go to the light. I keep praying.

Labor Day weekend is soon here. Did I say, soon? Seems like this has been going on for years! It's been three months. My birthday is usually over Labor Day weekend. My family always made a big deal out of each one of our birthdays. How much does mom remember? Does she know what date this is? That it is my birthday? She has not mentioned it. How much do they retain? She still has severe pain in her paralyzed leg, but her headaches have lessened. We have talks. She tells me to get on with my life. Right! She is my life.

My friends who were with us at the casino, Steve and Kirsten, make plans to take me out of town, up north to cool country, just to get away for the long weekend. I tell mom I am going out of town, which she encouraged me to do, but didn't remind her it was my birthday. I am packing to leave on Friday afternoon and you guessed it! The phone rings, informing me I have to move mom by Tuesday. Don't forget, Monday is a holiday. Again I ask, why do they have to wait until late in the afternoon, especially on a Friday, to give you a two day notice?

I explained I was leaving shortly to go out of town for the long weekend and wouldn't even be back until Tuesday. I begged the Director to give me until at least Friday. She agreed to Thursday. Really, what would happen in one day? I decided to go on my trip anyway to relax, enjoy and put worries on hold for a few days. I told mom once again I was leaving for a few days, but when I got back I was going to move her into a new home. She was thrilled!.

The nursing home she was in was nothing more than a glorified hospital and she wanted out. I had learned this from my father, a few others and now my mother. They always want to go home. I think they feel like they would be safer, more secure, if they were in their own environment but not able to fully comprehend the care they need. I decide to keep my plans and go away for a few days, to try and put my worries on hold. Easier said than done.

I return home and of course the first thing I do is visit mom. I went with two mutual friends of ours, who graciously had bought me a birthday cake and wanted to share it with me and mom. She was even thoughtful enough to bring a birthday card to have mom sign and give to me. Mom had remembered and was extremely grateful to our friend. Mom felt so ashamed she could not do this for me. As I cut the cake and tears are flowing from all around, I invite the caretakers in to celebrate with us letting all know it was my birthday. They said they already knew, as that was all mom had talked about over the weekend. So that answers that question, they do retain knowledge from the past. Now for the final battle.

The Hunt Resumed
Part 2

After returning home, I called Becky, my head hunter and let her know the situation. I told her the homes that were my first, second and third choices. Remember, I got smart enough to plan ahead? Right. All the homes we had decided in advance would be good choices were already full to their capacity.

I go to the nursing home Director, whom I had talked with before to explain the situation, begging for a one week continuance so I could find a proper home for mom. This time she was not budging and I was too emotionally worn out to fight anymore. I was told that if I didn't have her out by Friday, starting Saturday, the cost would be $190 a day. I wondered if that included doing her laundry!

Thank God I have a real life Angel as a head hunter. Becky works triple time to find me a place before Friday. Because she is so caring, she usually likes to visit the homes ahead of time to make sure they are going to be a good fit for her clients. We didn't have that kind of time luxury. She knew I was psychic and

99

didn't have an issue with that. She gave me full permission to use my instincts on making the correct choice. Bless her heart.

She did have six places scheduled for us to see. The first one we visited had a big Angel statue greeting us as soon as we walked into the door. Home! But we visited all of them. Some had such a bad feeling, that as soon as we drove up to the house, I said "NO", so we didn't even waste our time going in. We eventually went back to the "Angel house" and negotiated price, yes you can do that, and arranged to move mom on that Friday. (Please note, just like renting anywhere they also require a deposit. In most cases that is refundable if you don't move them or they pass. Make sure you go over the whole contract with anywhere you place your loved one. Very important) Mom loved it! Yea!

Unfortunately, the next day she became worse. And the day after that even worse, which of course was a Sunday. By Monday, Hospice was called to evaluate her. She was moved that afternoon into hospice. Now let's think back. Mom is 87 and frail. She suffered a stroke in June, and it is now September. She has been moved including air evacuated from the casino, six times in three months. I don't even move that often and I am in good health. In my mind I'm thinking this is it, right? If she is moved into hospice she has only a few days, weeks at most to live. Wrong again.

Hospice will not do anything to sustain life, such as any kind of life support. Their job is to make individuals as comfortable as possible, both in their surroundings and through medication. They do not force them to eat, but will administer IV's if needed to administer medication. While on the medications, mom developed a bladder infection, which they treated.

I found out she was on about 7-8 medications, which I addressed with hospice. Too much for a woman who hadn't taken any kind of prescription medication in years. Hospice adjusted her meds, and after two weeks they felt she was well enough to go back to her group home. I must admit, hospice was wonderful. They were very caring and heartfelt. Something I did not know is that a lot of people will not pass in a hospice facility. They will wait till they get back to their "home".

I am learning quickly that no one can tell you how much longer anyone has to live. That is strictly between the person and their higher self. Caretakers have great feelings about when their charges are about to go, within days, sometimes even hours, but until that time arrives, no one can help you. You must go on as if this will last for years. Now the thoughts go through my head, what about the money? How long will that last to sustain her in the home?

As I said earlier, Becky gave me the name of a guy who was very knowledgeable about VA benefits. Mom qualified as my father was a vet. This kind and generous man charged us nothing and used to give free seminars all over the country to educate people. Not only did he complete the whole process for me from start to finish, but he had mom's benefits in less than three months. Keep in mind, the money is retroactive, and the monthly benefits are quite substantial. There are many qualifications, first one being they must be on a self-pay. When they are in a nursing home receiving insurance benefits, they do not qualify.

Luckily, he knew all of the loop holes. As in my mom's case, once she went into the private home she had to pay out of her pocket as insurance does not cover this. That was when she qualified. I feel this is very sad. These veterans fought for their country, but to receive benefits is extremely difficult. But also be advised, there are people out there who will do this for you and charge a lot of money for their services, so just be careful. This kind, generous, caring man was a gift sent to me by God. I have no doubt. What will I learn tomorrow?

Onward

I am feeling good about myself. I have learned a lot. I keep doing everything humanly possible for my mom's best interest, but now I am turning everything over to God. I keep asking to help her and me for our best and highest self. I am trusting, believing, and then releasing it all.

Mom continues to grow weaker. She is barely eating. I learn people can go one day to several months without eating and still survive. She seems happy, loves her caretakers, has kept her sense of humor, and is not complaining as much. I know she is still in pain, but I have this feeling she is giving up and trying to stay as positive as she can. Perhaps she is finally coming to terms with the life lessons she came here to learn and feeling more at peace with everything.

I know in my heart of hearts, one of the main reasons she keeps hanging on is because of me. When she looks me in the eyes, I feel her love, thankfulness, her life's completeness and forgiveness. I assure her regularly I will be fine. I have many friends who will take care of me.

I talk to her daily about deceased loved ones, colors, Angels, God, giving her reassurance. Who better to do this than me since I have the direct connection. However, trust me it is easier to help others, than those who are closest to you. When she first arrived in her "Angel" house, she constantly rang the bell for assistance all times of the day and night. She was always seeing demons, ghosts, and all sort of scary things.

One night Joe, a very close friend of ours, and I went to visit. I felt the presence of a dragon that appeared to me as a big demon, not there for good. Not only is Joe a close friend but he has become highly intuitive with his spiritual gifts after taking many of my classes. I closed my eyes and brought in the Angels and God to disperse of this entity. Joe and I have such a close spiritual bond that we were able to communicate without voicing words. He had felt this presence as well. He knew exactly what I was doing and together, although it took a little while, we succeeded in dispersing this negative entity.

Now mom is sleeping through the evening serenely. I feel she is making peace with the demons she has had in the past and finding comfort from the higher side. As I have done many times over the last few months, I question what keeps us from going to the other side? Are we scared, not done here, or afraid of leaving our loved ones behind? I just don't get it. I have seen the other side and trust me when I say this, it is not scary.

Remains

After we had placed my father in a nursing home, we learned about a center that will take the body after a person has passed under two conditions. First you must agree to be cremated. Our philosophy on this, once a person has passed it is their soul that travels forward, not the physical body, so neither my mother nor I had a problem with cremation. Second, you must agree to allow them to use any part of the body they can for either research or organ donation.

This center was so kind, caring, and understanding and spent time with us answering questions. If you agree to their terms, then they will transport the body, cremate it and deliver the remains to you free of charge. I never have understood why people spend thousands of dollars for a burial, but to each their own.

I told the center about my dad having Alzheimer's and wanted them to see if anyone could use his brain to help with further research. After calling around the country, they did find a lab in California that agreed to do this. Not only did we sign my dad up, but both my mom and I signed up as well. I have told many about this, and have had many others agree to this. Once my dad did pass, they couldn't have been nicer or more efficient. This memory is a huge relief for me now facing what is going to happen to my mom. I know in my heart of hearts that I have done everything humanly possible for the welfare of my mother. Still I question, is it enough? Am I overlooking something?

"The Call"

On Nov. 16, 2009, I received the "dreaded call." I have received this "call" on two other occasions; once for my brother, once for my father. I don't understand how caretakers know when the end is near, but trust me they do. In my situation, my loved ones were all at different facilities. My brother Eric was in the hospital, my dad was at a VA nursing home for Alzheimer's, and my mom was in a private group home. It doesn't matter where they work, caretakers all just know.

The cause of my father's passing was multiple heart attacks. I kept getting calls at work informing he had had another. I finally had a meeting with the head nurse, explaining I could not keep taking off time from work, nor putting my mother through this emotional state every day. We agreed she would only call me when she felt the time was near.

When I remember that call, it is like it happened yesterday. It came on Saturday morning, one of my busiest days, as I was selling new homes in a very booming real estate market. I picked up my mom and

107

drove to his "home." Dad was totally unresponsive, breathing heavily, bad color. I assured him verbally it was ok to go, how brave he had been, what a great life he had lived. It's déjà vu all over again. I had done the same thing for my brother and I hadn't even awakened into my spiritual gifts yet.

This time I lovingly tell my dad is time to be with Eric, the Angels and God. It is time to have fun again. Mom and I would take care of each other. Then I stood back and mentally helped him to connect to the higher powers. Mom told him the same thing assuring him we would be ok. He took in a deep breath and we thought that was going to be the end. But dad didn't pass until that evening. Eric passed in the evening as well. Everyone has a different opinion on this but personally, I don't want to be present, nor have I been when any of my loved ones have passed, not even my dogs.

The "call" came about my mother on a Monday morning. I drop everything and rush to be by her side. She does recognize me and once again I assure her it is ok to go to the light. I try to comfort her with talk of Angels, Eric, dad, her deceased loved ones, and that I would be ok. I tell her she will actually be able to communicate with me better on the other side, and she laughs. After spending many hours with her, I decide to leave. Many times our loved ones will not pass if you are present. I felt it best to do the unselfish thing and leave her to her own passing, knowing deep down this might take some time.

Turmoil

Now, just like thousands of times in the past five months, I question whether I am making the correct decision. Should I leave her or stay? What am I going to do if I leave? It is the middle of the day. Most of my friends work. I know I could have called them, but I don't want to bother them. After all, this could go on for a while, right?

I was so lost, dazed, confused, sad, and angry. You name it, I felt it. I went through all the emotions. I drove to her mobile home park, to seek comfort there from her neighbors, most of who are retired. Not one of them is at home. A friend of mine was working from home that day, so I sought comfort there for a bit. Finally I went home to wait for the last call.

The call did not come. Keep in mind both my father and brother passed the night we said it was ok to go. Not my mom. Being independent, stubborn, and with a "my way or the highway" attitude, decides she is not ready to go that day or the next day.

Day 2. Back over I go to be with her. She is so much worse, which I didn't think could be possible. Again I give her reassurance, comfort, but most of all, my love.

It's the end of the day again, now what do I do? Didn't have a clue where to go, I just knew I didn't want to go home. A little voice told me to go back to the mobile home park. Since I am on automatic pilot, I don't question, I just listen and obey. To no surprise of mine, all the neighbors were home! I spent several hours visiting with them seeking comfort, but now it is time to leave. Now what? Another voice tells me to go to the Eagles which is a private club much like a VFW or American legion, where we have been members for years. I can't believe I am being guided to go have a beer!

I run into a friend who loved my mother. He didn't know anything about my mom's condition for the past five months. We sat there and chatted and cried for a long time. He told me if I needed anything to call. I told him once she passed I was going to have a celebration of her life at my home and needed yard work done. He brought his whole team over, worked for hours and was offended when I offered to pay him.

Now what? I went to friend's house to hang out for a while. It is now 7 pm. I am a basket case. So I went back to see mom. Usually that is pretty late to visit as they are getting their people ready for bed. But they have now come to treat me as family and welcome me with open arms. She was worse and incoherent, but I knew she was aware of me being there.

I sat on the back porch with one of the caretakers to talk. More like vent. There is nothing else for me to do, so I come home. I am very angry. I start throwing things which is definitely not my nature. I don't want her to suffer. Why can't she just go? Please God take her. Let her be better again. Within 30 minutes I received the "call" she had passed. Thank you God!

Passing

I called four friends, Joe, Steve, Kirsten and Phyllis, all of whom came right over. We sat on my back patio and began to pray. As I mentioned, Joe has special "gifts" or abilities like myself so we tuned into mom, better known as channeling. We were both trying to help her get to the other side as quickly and effortlessly as possible. Mom appeared to both of us loud and clear, in typical mom fashion. In unison, Joe and I were both saying the same thing.

"Look, I can move my arm now, I can walk, I can dance." Then mom held up a can of beer very pleased with herself. Keep in mind both of us were seeing and saying the exact same thing at the exact same time! Was this another coincidence? I don't believe in coincidences. She was so happy and free. I felt so much comfort, peace, but most importantly, love.

I had received my answers, so I pulled out of my channeled state. Joe stayed in his to see if he could receive any more messages. Phyllis continued to pray. I was facing east, Steve and Kirsten were facing south. All of a sudden at the same exact time, we saw a huge flash of white light in the sky. Almost like lightening. Mind you, by now it is 11:30 p.m. in November. Phoenix seldom has any storms in November. I said in a stunned voice, did you guys see that? Is it lightning out here? I was amazed and surprised. Steve and Kirsten were asking the same thing, all of us with our mouths open, remarking that was the most incredible thing we had ever witnessed. Even my friends, who know me well, remarked if they hadn't seen it with their own eyes, they would never have believed it. I know in my heart of hearts, that was mom's affirmation and confirmation. She had arrived and was doing fine. Yeah, well what took you so long?

Preparations

Now we start planning for the funeral, although I never have liked the word funeral. I want to have a celebration of her new life, one without pain and suffering. My friends decided the sooner the better for me. Keep in mind; it is now Wednesday with the next weekend being Thanksgiving. I call her neighbors to see if there was any way to have the services in the club house at her mobile home park to make it easier for the folks there who wanted to attend.

 Within a matter of hours the plans were almost finalized. Her one neighbor arranged for the club house as well as a minister. He came over to my house to talk, as I didn't want the traditional ceremony. I told him my thoughts and feelings about the spiritual world and to my amazement, he was in total agreement. I told him I wanted to keep it upbeat, happy and fun, having people realize she was no longer in pain, as that would be what mom would have wanted. I'm telling you, this minister was sent to me straight from God and mom. He was perfect. He spent several hours with me and my good friend

Judy, capturing the true essence of mom so he could convey those images to everyone.

Many people wanted to speak about their memories of mom, but no one wanted to go first. I had to lead the way, which is exactly what mom had planned. I didn't sleep much the night before for many obvious reasons, but mainly what did mom want me to talk about? I talked about her trip to the zoo, where a tiger jumped on a fence and roared and she peed in her pants. Then many other fun filled loving times, ending of course with the story about the huge flash of white light. I could see in the eyes of everyone, even the non-believers that they had all understood!

Many others got up to convey their experiences with Margaret, mostly making everyone laugh behind their tears. This is the way mom would have wanted her celebration to go. Mind you not everyone would want this type of service, but I honored and respected who my mom was and what she would have wanted. I know she was up there, laughing, clapping and having a beer with us. She always did like parties. I had them write on the cake for the service, Mom May You Always Play with the Angels.

Even though I was brave and strong enough to speak at her "celebration" it still took its toll on me. After all, I am only human. Some say super human, but human none the less. After the services, I started feeling dizzy, light headed and felt my heart racing much like I had after visiting mom in the hospital the first day. Luckily for me some of our mutual friends that were there were nurses. Along with Joe, they sat me down until I was able to get my pulse rate and head back to normal; whatever passes for normal in these circumstances. Again I stress to you, do not be alone under these conditions. You might think you are strong and can "handle it" but you just never know.

After the clubhouse service, many of us came back to my house for another celebration. People came and went all night. I was on auto pilot. I know my friends were taking care of me, but honestly I don't remember much. Even though I know she is in a better place, I still can't believe she is truly gone. I did receive affirmation that she made it ok, but it all still seems so unreal. Is this really happening or has this all been just a dream? Will I ever wake up? How will I go on without any family?

I know my friends will watch over me, but I hate to burden anyone. What is going to happen to me now? I have given up most of my life to help mom for the past five months. There is no way at this point in time I can do readings and my real estate has been put on hold. What lies ahead of me as far as tying up loose ends on my mother's behalf? Legal issues? Bills, taxes, and the rest of the things in her home? Trying to get her home sold so I don't have to pay rent on the space any more. So many questions. So few answers. I try not to think and just live in the moment. How can I go on? I am all alone! I am truly the last soul standing.

Afterwards

Upon awakening the next morning, I feel great! Happy! Did I have a complete breakdown last night, and now am in a mental facility heavily sedated? No, I am in my own bed, in my own room, in my own house, alone, and I am OK! It is a release. I know mom is WELL taken care of now. No more suffering. I don't have to wait for either the dreaded call or any call where I have to handle some issue again. Don't get me wrong. I know there is still plenty to do, but not today. It's Saturday and everything can wait. I need time to get my brain functioning again.

I turn on TV and much to my surprise, the Ohio State Michigan football game, (big rivalry) is on! Yea and there is beer in the fridge. You would have thought I had died and gone to heaven. Does this sound cruel? Sorry, but that's how I felt. My family always watched this game together, so I know they were there with me. If I had been aware the game was on that day, yes I would have bet that Ohio State would win. Are you kidding me, with my whole family now on the other side, of course winning was going to be a no brainer, and it was. Miraculously, because I don't remember much, I made it through the whole weekend.

Luckily the next week I was busy with a real estate transaction, and this week only had three days in it because of Thanksgiving. Now how am I going to handle my first holiday and a big one at that, all alone? Yes, I had many invitations. People inviting me to their homes to be with their family (yeah right), or just friends, a cabin up north, or coming to my house and cook.

I appreciated all the invitations, but I really didn't want to be with anyone. I guess I just needed Marilyn time to process everything. Cry, laugh sleep, cook, drink; whatever I wanted when I wanted to in my time. Is this a healing or poor me pity party? I vote for healing. The last couple of years, mom and I had spent Thanksgiving mainly alone having fun. Cooking when we felt like it, laughing, drinking, watching TV, whatever our hearts felt like doing. That is what I wanted to do this year. Off to the store I went to get the smallest turkey I could find, potatoes, Stove Top stuffing, and a bottle of wine and I was all set. I made it through my first Thanksgiving without family. I even played golf the next day which was a huge release for me.

December

The whole month of December I was busy. Imagine that. This from a girl who had barely worked in six months. Not only did I have real estate transactions, but people were calling to schedule readings and classes. Thank you Angels for watching over and taking care of me. I love you!!! Now Christmas is upon me. I am receiving Christmas cards for mom. What do I do? Do I let people know she has passed? I can hardly face this yet, let alone respond to these people to let them know, so I elect to put these on ignore.

What is going on in my brain constantly is how will I get through Christmas without any family? It's a big question. In over 50 some years, I was never apart from my parents at Christmas. Dad has been gone five years now, but mom and I have spent all the Christmases together. What am I going to do? This holiday I do not want to spend alone but I'm not sure if I can handle it at a friend's house with their family.

Thankfully, my friends Steve and Kirsten suggest we go to Laughlin, NV to gamble. Perfect. This is what other friends of mine along with my parents did the first year after I had left my husband. Only people with no families or who didn't care about Christmas would spend it in a casino, right? I will have my friends with me in case I have a break down, but I won't have to think or do anything at least for a few days. It will be a pure escape from it all. Only requirement is to eat, drink, gamble and be merry! We did have a good time, but I knew in the back of my head I would have to come back to reality. Why can't I just hit one of the big jackpots and escape from reality forever? The Angels of course had other plans for me.

Of course the next week is New Year's Eve, no biggie because I have spent many eve's without my mom. I had broken up with my boyfriend of six years just two months prior to mom's stroke. It just never ends. Again the Angels watch over me. The day after we get back from Laughlin, I get sick. In bed I go. What a relief this is. Can I stay here forever? NO! There are things that cannot wait.

Stuff

I can't sell her mobile home. I can't afford to keep paying the rent. I have made numerous attempts to contact the management company to see if they would work with me but never received a return phone call. I don't know all the legal ramifications, but I am led to believe that either I pay the rent, sign the deed over to management, or be sued. I never investigated this, whether they could sue me, even though everything was in my mother's name, but I didn't have it in me to fight with anyone anymore. So I had to go into the office, emotionally and physically drained, and sign the deed over to the management so they can now have her home at no cost to them. Was this the correct thing to do? I had many opinions from well-meaning people, but I could no longer handle any more conflicts. I just wanted everything to be over and go away.

Now comes the hardest part. Go back to her home one more time and finish sorting through all of her "stuff"; her personal belongings, clothes, jewelry, bathroom items, Christmas items, and all of the knickknacks that meant so much to her. There are piles and piles of stuff. I have spent an entire week loading up my SUV with the things I could not bear to part with at this time, crying my eyes out. Taking what I want, and giving the rest to a charity for people trying to get back on their feet. Hopefully, these people made good use of her things.

Now my house is on over flow. I can barely park my car in the garage, and a spare bedroom I use as an office is so crowded. There is only a tiny space I created so I can at least get to my computer. I have to get to my computer as my life saver at this time is playing spider solitaire. Still I feel sick. Doesn't anyone understand, or care for that matter? All I want to do is crawl into bed, pull the covers over my head and make it all go away. Yet the bills keep rolling in. Well-wishers keep calling, or emailing. Christmas cards keep coming for Margaret. Everyone thinks I am fine, because I am not showing or expressing my true emotions. That would show weakness, right? I am supposed to be a strong person.

Now it is New Year's Eve and still sick. I stay home and celebrate by myself. What will the next year bring? More loneliness I would think. Who is going to be here to help me, guide me, and talk to me? It's New Year's Eve so it is ok to drink alcohol, right. As much as I want since I am not driving and no one is around to hear my depression. I have a complete, major crying breakdown. I guess that's why they tell you depression and alcohol do not mix. Right now I just don't care. I go to bed and in my heart of hearts, hope I never wake up.

New Year

I wake up the next day extremely dizzy. Wonder why? I can barely make it to the bathroom. Everything is spinning so badly. Is it from the alcohol, depression, or am I having a stroke, heart attack? Don't care. I make it back to my blessed bed, to welcome the comforting sleep. I can sleep forever. Hope I never wake up. I just want to be with my family. This goes on for over a month. Yes I know I have things to do, but sleep is much more comforting. Someone else handles things. I just don't care and I'm still looking, or more like craving, for the day I never wake up.

Friends are getting mad at me because I am not behaving the way they think I should. (How would that be?) I am not returning phone calls, emails or visiting. Leave me alone everyone. Can't you see I am sick? I know they are concerned but right now I just don't care. If you are truly my friend, you will understand and leave me alone. Let me add right here, I would never do that to a friend, but I am not thinking coherently at this time. If you are truly my friend, you will still be here when I wake up, if I ever do. If I never wake up, that means I have passed and can be with my whole family again, including all of the animals I have had as pets over the years. Now that would be wonderful! I would never have to worry about handling anymore "stuff." Yes I understand my friends would miss me, but that would soon pass, as they still all have family left here to take care of them. I have no one. Obviously, God and His band of Angels had bigger plans for me. (Remember God never gives you more than you can handle)

Waking Up

Upon awakening one morning, when I am not dreading waking up as much, a thought occurred to me. I was like an ostrich. I can keep burying my head in the sand with my butt sticking up in the air, letting people keep kicking it, or I can pull my head out of the sand and start standing on my own two feet. Now where did this come from? I don't even know anything about the habits of ostriches and I am a rational person! (If you believe that I was rational at this time in my life, I will sell you swamp land in AZ!) It was divine intervention. It is what I needed to understand to pull my big girl pants up and start getting on with my life!

I started allowing people to return into my life. Old friends started coming back and I was now out in public making new friends. My relationships begin to grow stronger as I do! I now realize the stuff left behind, is just "stuff". It still has to be dealt with, but I take it one day at a time. As the old saying goes, Rome wasn't built in a day. Whatever I can deal with today is what I will accomplish.

As I am handling things, I am growing emotionally stronger as well. I realize if I need to take a day off to sleep, that is ok. We all heal in different ways at different speeds. How one person heals, whether from a physical injury or mental, it all happens in different times. What worked well for one person, might not work for you. I am learning there are no rules for this disease called depression. I am discovering, the more you can do to handle the issues that need to be dealt with, the faster you heal.

Handling

I begin to handle. For several months, I have had a whole box filled with all of her bills lying on my kitchen table. I start going through all of them. What is owed and how I am going to pay the remainder. Coming from the medical field, I decide to call to explain she has passed. Fortunately a friend of a friend suggested sending the bills back with a letter stating this instead of calling. This turned out to be great advice. Do you know what it is like to try and call a doctor's office these days to actually talk to someone? I make a copy of her death certificate, insurance cards and a generic letter, put these all in an envelope with the appropriate bill, and sent them off.

I had even received a bill from the TV satellite provider, which I had cancelled six months prior, for $70. After spending over an hour on the phone, explaining mom had a stroke and passed five months later, they still wanted the money because she still had 1 1/2 years remaining on her contract. After much debate and several supervisors later, they agreed not to hurt her credit, if I returned the receivers along with a copy of her death certificate. I explained I did not have access to her home anymore but would be happy to give them the phone number to the management company that now owns the home. They cannot make phone calls. Do you really think she cares about her credit? Again, I am so thankful I do not have a real job. How do people handle all of this along with working a full time job and dealing with children and spouses?

I continually receive a minimum of 20-30 advertisements a week from all the casinos Margaret frequented. I call them all to ask them to please stop. It is a daily reminder of mom and her life. I am trying to put these memories, at least for now, on a back burner of my brain. I am told that the only way to have them discontinue with these is with her written permission! Say what? How am I supposed to do that? I do believe in divine intervention, but really? I explain I need to heal and this isn't helping. I was instructed to send her death certificate, but it would be up to a supervisor to determine whether they would discontinue these ads. What does the supervisor have to determine. That she is really dead?

These are just a few examples of the things I dealt with for hours a day, week after week to handle the "stuff," to help me heal. Thank goodness no one has called to schedule an Angel reading, or is it? I need money to live on and my readings are my livelihood. But can I help others, when I am barely helping myself?

Moving On

The first month of the New Year is almost gone. I have sorted through many things both on a physical and emotional level. I am not sleeping as much and getting out in public more, but I seem to have no direction, no focus, no guidance. Or is it I am not listening?

Mentally at this time I know I cannot do my Angel work and I feel in my heart of hearts, I am done with real estate. Now what? I do need money to live on. I am not independently wealthy. Mom didn't leave much behind. I keep telling everyone even to this day, if mom would have left me as much money as she did Kleenex, I would never have to worry about money again!

I hear a little voice in my ear say write a book! After laughing hysterically, at least I am laughing now, I proceed to argue. Say what? Write a book. I did say while I was going through those five months, after the dust settles, I was going to write a book. The problem then was the dust never settled. I continue to argue

131

with that voice, which I know are the Angels guiding me ever so gently on to a higher path.

So I defend myself by asking "now how am I going to do that?" The voice says to me "look to your left." There on the couch sat a catalog from a community college where I have taken several classes over the years. Pick it up. So I thumb through it. There isn't anything about writing a book. See I told you. Thumb through the back pages. And there it was. On one of the very back pages was a class being offered within the next week. It was called *How to write your book in 30 days or less*. It was 3 ½ hours and only $19. I am being guided by my Angels so how could I lose? My life completely turned around that night.

I begin to sleep even less, because I now have a purpose, a direction. I begin to feel excited about life again. I signed up to take the instructor's ten day book writing retreat in beautiful Sedona, Arizona, the land of Angels. Imagine. There were 30 people there from all over the world. I write this book by hand in less than three days. I also started another book. The writing of this book released so many feelings that were still lying deep and buried. Feelings that I did not want to deal with. I am now finding release and purpose. I have so many good people in my life right now. I even started playing golf again.

I still have issues to deal with, but now I am getting stronger to be able to handle them without feeling like a ball and chain are wrapped around my body. I am back to taking my daily walks. Trust it is true what they say. Exercise is a good stress reliever. People are calling me all the time to receive readings!

I know I still have a long way to go, but at least now I am moving in a forward direction with powerful positive energy to help me survive without my family. I can't wait to see what directions the Angels and God take me.

The Book

My intentions for writing this book are to help anyone out there who is dealing with a loved one with any kind of debilitating disease or condition. I know how dumb struck I felt when my mother suffered her stroke and the events that took place before her passing, even given my vast knowledge of medical practices and personal experiences with my brother's and father's diseases.

I sincerely want to enlighten everyone, with or without previous knowledge, to all of the help that is available to you. I have only named a few that I personally encountered, but if this can help just one person, then I feel blessed. If that person shares with one other person, then I am doubly blessed! If these reach millions who receive help, then everything I have gone through, not to mention the pain and suffering my loved ones went through, will not have been in vain.

The many different resources that I have offered you are also there for you. If they can't help you ask them if they know of someone who can. Keep asking until you receive the help you need. Don't let depression, frustration, or anger block your way.

Please don't make the mistake I did, thinking this will never happen to you or your loved ones. I always felt, or probably hoped, that mom would just pass quietly in her sleep one day as her father did. You do not know what lies ahead for you or your loved ones. You can ask your higher source for anything you want. You have free will to change anything in your life. All you have to do is ask. But you cannot change someone else's life path. You can only be there for them to offer love, comfort, and protection.

I highly suggest you start preparing now, no matter your circumstance. It doesn't have to be a disease or be an old age. Any type of transportation, with an engine can be fatal in a mini second. Even just falling down can have a long term impact. Do research. With the internet it is now much easier and less time consuming. Ask friends, read books, go to support groups.

You don't know what lies ahead for you or your loved ones, but certain things you can make sure about now. Medical insurance, what is covered and what is not. The little helicopter ride mom had to the hospital was over $17,000. Her hospital bill alone for two weeks was over $100,000. Understand now what portion you are responsible for, because you will continue to receive billing until it is all cleared. Some people see a bill and think they have to pay it. Does your insurance provide for long term care? Do you need a supplemental? What medication are you currently taking and what are you allergic to? Write all of this down and carry it with you. Also make sure others have copies.

Understand your financial situation and have the proper people in place knowing all of your intentions. How will your children be taken care of? It truly upsets me when I see something happen to an elderly couple, who have worked and saved for years. Then something happens to their significant other, and the healthy one can go bankrupt because they had not properly planned.

Seek advice from an attorney or a financial advisor while you are still healthy and sound to understand your options. Many will allow a 60 minute consultation at no charge. Ask about a will and living trust, to see what is better for you. Do you want to be on life support? If not make sure you have this document legalized and everyone knows where it is. If you do not provide a legal DNR, the medical people have no choice but to try to keep you alive. Once you have this in place make copies to give to your loved ones and let everyone know where all your legal documents are.

Talk to your doctor or other people you know in the medical field. Do you want to be buried or cremated? Donate organs? If cremation and organ donation are acceptable, research organizations like my family did that have the whole body donor program and will handle the remains at no charge.

Talk to your insurance agent. Seek advice from professionals, not your friends. Friends mean well, but everyone has their own opinion, and what worked for them might not work for you.

What type of funeral service do you want? Let your loved ones know. I know this is painful to discuss. I never could get my parents to commit to anything. Trust me the only thing in life that you are 100% guaranteed, if you are born, you will die. Although, I don't like to say die, we pass to go home. Designate who you want to be in charge of this and let others know of your intentions.

Finally, and this is the important one, forgive so you have no guilt. Everyone has had someone make them mad and you have made someone else mad in your lifetime. This is life. If you have not forgiven a loved one for whatever reason, there is no time like the present to do so. I can't tell you how many readings I have done helping people forgive and release their guilt. You never know when someone is going to pass. So if there is anyone in your life, no matter whom they are, or what the circumstance was, make amends, do it now.

If you feel the need to reach out and communicate with them, whether that would entail a phone call, email, card, letter, seeking help from a professional or if you need to make the peace in another way by asking Angels for help or meditating to forgive, now is the time. Do this for yourself. If something would have happened to my mom during one of our many fights and she had passed while we were on a no speaking basis, I truly do not know how I would feel today.

I have no regrets about my life with my family. Anything bad that has happened, I have forgiven. I know in my heart of hearts, I have done everything I could have done for all of them with no regrets, and I know they know that as well. We all carry that love in our hearts whether they are here on this earth plane with me or not.

It is that forgiveness, no guilt, and love that inspired me to create this book and now complete it. And in doing so my heart now knows I am not the last soul standing.

In Light!

Addendum

Preparing for Approaching Death

(Reprinted with the permission of the author North Central Florida Hospice, Inc.)

When a person enters the final stage of the dying process, two different dynamics are at work which are closely interrelated and interdependent. On the physical plane, the body begins the final process of shutting down, which will end when all the physical systems cease to function. Usually this is an orderly and un-dramatic progressive series of physical changes which are not medical emergencies requiring invasive interventions. These physical changes are a normal, natural way in which the body prepares itself to stop, and the most appropriate kinds of responses are comfort enhancing measures.

The other dynamic of the dying process at work is on the emotional-spiritual-mental plane, and is a different kind of process. The spirit of the dying person begins the final process of release from the body, its immediate environment, and all attachments. This release also tends to follow its own priorities, which may include the resolution of whatever is unfinished of a practical nature and reception of permission to "let go" from family members. These events are the normal, natural way in which the spirit prepares to move from this existence into the next dimension of life. The most appropriate kinds of responses to the emotional-spiritual-mental changes are those which support and encourage this release and transition.

When a person's body is ready and wanting to stop, but the person is still unresolved or un-reconciled over some important issue or with some significant relationship, he or she may tend to linger in order to finish whatever needs finishing even though he or she may be uncomfortable or debilitated. On the other hand, when a person is emotionally-spiritually-mentally resolved and ready for this release, but his or her body has not completed its final physical shut down, the person will continue to live until that shut down process ceases.

The experience we call death occurs when the body completes its natural process of shutting down, and when the spirit completes its natural process of reconciling and finishing. These two processes need to happen in a way appropriate and unique to the values, beliefs, and lifestyle of the dying person.

Therefore, as you seek to prepare yourself as this event approaches, the members of your Hospice care team want you to know what to expect and how to respond in ways that will help your loved one accomplish this transition with support, understanding, and ease. This is the great gift of love you have to offer your loved one as this moment approaches.

The emotional-spiritual-mental and physical signs and symptoms of impending death which follow are offered to help you understand the natural kinds of things which may happen and how you can respond appropriately. Not all these signs and symptoms will occur with every person, nor will they occur in this particular sequence. Each person is unique and needs to do things in his or her own way. This is not the time to try to change your loved one, but the time to give full acceptance, support, and comfort.

The following signs and symptoms described are indicative of how the body prepares itself for the final stage of life.

Coolness
The person's hands and arms, feet and then legs may be increasingly cool to the touch, and at the same time the color of the skin may change. This a normal indication that the circulation of blood is decreasing to the body's extremities and being reserved for the most vital organs. Keep the person warm with a blanket, but do not use one that is electric.

Sleeping

The person may spend an increasing amount of time sleeping, and appear to be uncommunicative or unresponsive and at times be difficult to arouse. This normal change is due in part to changes in the metabolism of the body. Sit with your loved one, hold his or her hand, but do not shake it or speak loudly. Speak softly and naturally. Plan to spend time with your loved one during those times when he or she seems most alert or awake. Do not talk about the person in the person's presence. Speak to him or her directly as you normally would, even though there may be no response. Never assume the person cannot hear; hearing is the last of the senses to be lost.

Disorientation

The person may seem to be confused about the time, place, and identity of people surrounding him or her including close and familiar people. This is also due in part to the metabolism changes. Identify yourself by name before you speak rather than to ask the person to guess who you are. Speak softly, clearly, and truthfully when you need to communicate something important for the patient's comfort, such as, It is time to take your medication, and explain the reason for the communication, such as, so you won't begin to hurt. Do not use this method to try to manipulate the patient to meet your needs.

Incontinence

The person may lose control of urine and/or bowel matter as the muscles in that area begin to relax. Discuss with your Hospice nurse what can be done to protect the bed and keep your loved one clean and comfortable.

Congestion

The person may have gurgling sounds coming from his or her chest as though marbles were rolling around inside these sounds may become very loud. This normal change is due to the decrease of fluid intake and an inability to cough up normal secretions. Suctioning usually only increases the secretions and causes sharp discomfort. Gently turn the person s head to the side and allow gravity to drain the secretions. You may also gently wipe the mouth with a moist cloth. The sound of the congestion does not indicate the onset of severe or new pain.

Restlessness

The person may make restless and repetitive motions such as pulling at bed linen or clothing. This often happens and is due in part to the decrease in oxygen circulation to the brain and to metabolism changes. Do not interfere with or try to restrain such motions. To have a calming effect, speak in a quiet, natural way, lightly massage the forehead, read to the person, or play some soothing music.

Urine Decrease
The person's urine output normally decreases and may become tea colored referred to as concentrated urine. This is due to the decreased fluid intake as well as decrease in circulation through the kidneys. Consult with your Hospice nurse to determine whether there may be a need to insert or irrigate a catheter.

Fluid and Food Decrease
The person may have a decrease in appetite and thirst, wanting little or no food or fluid. The body will naturally begin to conserve energy which is expended on these tasks. Do not try to force food or drink into the person, or try to use guilt to manipulate them into eating or drinking something. To do this only makes the person much more uncomfortable. Small chips of ice, frozen Gatorade or juice may be refreshing in the mouth. If the person is able to swallow, fluids may be given in small amounts by syringe (ask the Hospice nurse for guidance). Glycerin swabs may help keep the mouth and lips moist and comfortable. A cool, moist washcloth on the forehead may also increase physical comfort.

Breathing Pattern Change
The person s regular breathing pattern may change with the onset of a different breathing pace. A particular pattern consists of breathing irregularly, i.e., shallow breaths with periods of no breathing of five to thirty seconds and up to a full minute. This is called Cheyne-Stokes breathing. The person may also experience periods of rapid shallow pant-like breathing. These patterns are very common and indicate decrease in circulation in the internal organs. Elevating the head, and/or turning the person onto his or her side may bring comfort. Hold your loved one's hand. Speak gently.

Normal Emotional, Spiritual, and Mental Signs and Symptoms with Appropriate Responses

Withdrawal
The person may seem unresponsive, withdrawn, or in a comatose-like state. This indicates preparation for release, a detaching from surroundings and relationships, and a beginning

of letting go. Since hearing remains all the way to the end, speak to your loved one in your normal tone of voice, identifying yourself by name when you speak, hold his or her hand, and say whatever you need to say that will help the person let go.

Vision-like experiences
The person may speak or claim to have spoken to persons who have already died, or to see or have seen places not presently accessible or visible to you. This does not indicate an hallucination or a drug reaction. The person is beginning to detach from this life and is being prepared for the transition so it will not be frightening. Do not contradict, explain away, belittle or argue about what the person claims to have seen or heard. Just because you cannot see or hear it does not mean it is not real to your loved one. Affirm his or her experience. They are normal and common. If they frighten your loved one, explain that they are normal occurrences.

Restlessness
The person may perform repetitive and restless tasks. This may in part indicate that something still unresolved or unfinished is disturbing him or her, and prevents him or her from letting go. Your Hospice team members will assist you in identifying what may be happening, and help you find ways to help the person find release from the tension or fear. Other things which may be helpful in calming the person are to recall a favorite place the person enjoyed, a favorite experience, read something comforting, play music, and give assurance that it is OK to let go.

Fluid and Food Decrease
When the person may want little or no fluid or food; this may indicate readiness for the final shut down. Do not try to force food or fluid. You may help your loved one by giving permission to let go whenever he or she is ready. At the same time affirm the person s ongoing value to you and the good you will carry forward into your life that you received from him or her.

Decreased Socialization
The person may only want to be with a very few or even just one person. This is a sign of preparation for release and affirms from whom the support is most needed in order to make the appropriate transition. If you are not part of this inner circle at the end, it does not mean you are not loved or are unimportant. It means you have already fulfilled your task with your loved one, and it is the time for you to say Good-bye. If you are part of

145

the final inner circle of support, the person needs your affirmation, support, and permission.

Unusual communication
The person may make a seemingly out of character or non sequitur statement, gesture, or request. This indicates that he or she is ready to say Good-bye and is testing you to see if you are ready to let him or her go. Accept the moment as a beautiful gift when it is offered. Kiss, hug, hold, cry, and say whatever you most need to say.

Giving Permission
Giving permission to your loved one to let go, without making him or her guilty for leaving or trying to keep him or her with you to meet your own needs, can be difficult. A dying person will normally try to hold on, even though it brings prolonged discomfort, in order to be sure those who are going to be left behind will be all right. Therefore, your ability to release the dying person from this concern and give him or her assurance that it is all right to let go whenever he or she is ready is one of the greatest gifts you have to give your loved one at this time.

Saying Good-bye
When the person is ready to die and you are able to let go, then is the time to say, Good-bye. Saying Good-bye is your final gift of love to your loved one, for it achieves closure and makes the final release possible. It may be helpful to lay in bed and hold the person, or to take his or her hand and then say everything you need to say.

It may be as simple as saying, I love you. It may include recounting favorite memories, places, and activities you shared. It may include saying, I 'm sorry for whatever I contributed to any tension or difficulties in our relationship. It may also include saying, Thank you for...

Tears are a normal and natural part of saying, Good-bye. Tears do not need to be hidden from your loved one or apologized for. Tears express your love and help you to let go.

How Will You Know When Death Has Occurred?
Although you may be prepared for the death process, you may not be prepared for the actual death moment. It may be helpful for you and your family to think about and discuss what you would do if you were the one present at the death moment. The

death of a hospice patient is not an emergency. Nothing must be done immediately.

The signs of death include such things as no breathing, no heartbeat, release of bowel and bladder, no response, eyelids slightly open, pupils enlarged, eyes fixed on a certain spot, no blinking, jaw relaxed and mouth slightly open. A hospice nurse will come to assist you if needed or desired. If not, phone support is available.

The body does not have to be moved until you are ready. If the family wants to assist in preparing the body by bathing or dressing, that may be done. Call the funeral home when you are ready to have the body moved, and identify the person as a Hospice patient. The police do not need to be called. The Hospice nurse will notify the physician.

Thank you

We of Hospice thank you for the privilege of assisting you with the care of your loved one. We salute you for all you have done to surround your loved one with understanding care, to provide your loved one with comfort and calm, and to enable your loved one to leave this world with a special sense of peace and love.

You have given your loved one one of the most wonderful, beautiful, and sensitive gifts we humans have to offer, and in giving that gift have given yourself a wonderful gift as well.

About the Author

Marilyn Poscic is a nationally known, Angel Messenger and Medium, Psychic Counselor and Educator. She assists hundreds of people each year in finding their own spiritual guidance by connecting them to their inner truth.

Marilyn helps to reveal the lessons we are here to learn, by expanding our ability to recognize, hear and heed our Angels and other Spiritual Guides, including deceased loved ones. She consistently brings greater personal awareness, comfort, healing and closure to those who experience her teaching and messages.

A spiritual teacher with the ability to counsel others to help them awaken to their own spiritual gifts and divine life purpose, Marilyn not only shares the messages she receives but also gives people the confidence and capability to do this on their own by attending her classes. Marilyn enables us to reach a better balance between our human and spiritual side and to achieve a clearer understanding of the lessons we must learn in this life.

Her only goal is to achieve an abundance of happiness, harmony, wellness, and wealth for all by creating a better feeling of love, peace and joy within everyone.

She is currently at work on her second book, *Time, Reason and Season,* a true story based on her own spiritual awakening.

If you are interested in receiving Marilyn's newsletter to stay in touch with her and with her angels please email her at <u>Marilyn@marilynposcic.com</u>

Marilyn would also be happy to autograph your book. Send her an email and she'll let you know how to make that happen.

If you would like to have an angel reading (these can be done over the phone) email Marilyn at <u>Marilyn@marilynposcic.com</u>

For more information and a schedule of her classes please visit her website at: <u>www.marilynposcic.com</u> or email her at <u>Marilyn@marilynposcic.com</u>

Made in the USA
San Bernardino, CA
22 October 2014